"Functional medicine—root cause medicine, as it's sometimes called—is your road map to freedom and wellness. For women's specific concerns, functional medicine shines particularly brightly. Carrie Levine holds your hand through the many questions you've likely had (or may have) over your health journey and guides you to answers that make sense and work. Well-illustrated with case examples from her own clinical practice, this book is an essential reference for women who want to be hopeful and empowered in their health care."

**KARA FITZGERALD**, ND, IFMCP, physician, clinical researcher, author of *Younger You*

"As a seasoned women's health practitioner, Carrie Levine distills complex scientific concepts into accessible next steps to heal your body, mind, and spirit. Levine is gifted in her ability to voice the collective wisdom of diverse women, backed by science and informed by intuition. This is a must-read for any woman looking to live a healthier life."

**ELLEN VORA**, MD, author of *The Anatomy of Anxiety*

"Carrie Levine's book is practical and accessible, like the auntie I wish I had as I was learning about my own body as a woman. Her wisdom and knowledge are applicable to any age and demystify some of the myths or misbeliefs many of us were taught. This is a handbook you will keep close by for years to come."

**ALEXANDRA ROXO**, bestselling author of *F*ck like a Goddess: Heal Yourself. Reclaim Your Voice. Stand in Your Power.*

"*Whole Woman Health* gives us specific direction as to how we can greatly improve our physical health while nourishing our mind and spirit. Using case studies, Carrie Levine details the personalized way she uncovers root cause issues of imbalance and disease as a functional medicine practitioner. She outlines specific tests used to discover core issues and reveals how she uses diet, lifestyle, medications, and supplements to optimize health. Levine also includes a questionnaire to help you discover where some of your issues may lie. If you want to make a change and know more about your own body and health, read, then apply the wisdom in this book."

**ELIZABETH LIPSKI**, PhD, CNS, IFMCP, author of *Digestive Wellness* and founder of Innovative Healing

whole
woman
health

A GUIDE
TO CREATING
WELLNESS
FOR ANY AGE
AND STAGE

CARRIE E. LEVINE, CNM

# whole woman health

PAGE TWO

Cataloguing in publication information is
available from Library and Archives Canada.
ISBN 978-1-77458-303-6 (paperback)
ISBN 978-1-77458-304-3 (ebook)

Page Two
pagetwo.com

Edited by Kendra Ward
Copyedited by Rachel Ironstone
Proofread by Steph VanderMeulen
Cover and interior design by Fiona Lee

carrielevine.com

*For women—all shapes, colors, sizes, and nationalities*

· · · · · · · · · · · · · · · · ·

Although this book uses the nouns "woman" and "women," the author recognizes that not all people with female anatomy identify as women. The information in this book is intended for and inclusive of anyone with female anatomy, regardless of their gender identity.

# Contents

· · · · · · · · · · · · · · · · ·

# Introduction
# Embarking on a Path
# to Wholeness

. . . . . . . . . . . . . .

WHEN THE idea of writing an introductory guide to functional medicine for women first began to take form in my mind, I thought of the many women who have come to see me over the years. Each has her own unique health issue (or issues), her own strengths, and her own individualized path toward wholeness ahead of her. Many face serious disease and feel vulnerable and afraid, concerned with making good decisions about their health, while also needing support, care, and protection. Making giant decisions when we feel vulnerable is challenging.

I thought of one woman I took care of, Jenn, who told me a story about trying to decide on treatment when she was diagnosed with breast cancer. At the time, she was a single working mother with an eight-year-old daughter. She described how difficult it had been for her to think "clearly" under those circumstances. She lamented the choices she would have made differently had she known then what she learned when we started working together. Lamenting is an unavoidable part of the human experience, but sometimes a better job could be done, *in the moment*, of supporting, caring, and protecting people who are vulnerable.

I thought of Stacey, who described herself as being in "desperate" need of sleep. For the three months prior to our meeting, she'd skipped her period, had hot flashes, experienced vaginal dryness, and had not gotten more than four hours of sleep a night. She had tried acupuncture, valerian, and melatonin. She ran a seasonal business, and despite it being the busy time of year, she did not feel particularly stressed. She said she had good sleep hygiene—going to bed at the same time every night, waking up at the same time every morning, staying off screens before bed, and sleeping in a dark, cool room. Still, she was unable to sleep. We talked about the potential benefits of magnesium threonate, phosphatidyl serine, and tart cherry juice as we waited for the results of her hormone test. We discussed herbs that might support hormone balance and the circumstances under which she may opt to try hormone therapy.

I reflected on when I read *Perfect Madness: Motherhood in the Age of Anxiety* by Judith Warner. At the time, I was a breastfeeding mom, tending births as a midwife, horrifically sleep deprived, and not a very happy person. The message I took from her book was that kids need their mothers to be happy. It doesn't matter if we work full-time or part-time, if kids go to daycare or have a nanny. What they need is for *us* to be happy. And I thought to myself, "How am I supposed to know what I need to be happy? I haven't slept through a night in four years. I'm swinging from rung to rung to keep my job and my home afloat..." There was little time for reflection, let alone exploration. It felt unrealistic to think I could discern in those circumstances what I needed to be healthy. When I finally did figure it out, when the kids were a little bit older and I'd had a night or two of solid sleep, I *was* happier and healthier, and my family was too.

More and more, we are charged "to know our own truth," "to stand in our power," and "to trust our innate wisdom." For many of us, knowing our truth is harder than it sounds, as is standing in our power when we are vulnerable and afraid or in the middle of a personal catastrophe. Seeking care, support, and protection, we too often hand over our power, or are required to hand over our power, to health professionals. We learn to distrust what we know to be true for ourselves, or our personal experience is disregarded by the person from whom we seek help.

While innate wisdom serves as an invaluable compass, frankly, it is not always accurate or enough. Women say to me, "I know my body, and I would know if something was wrong." Except when we don't. Why wouldn't we avail ourselves of the science of the time? What harm is there in integrating innate wisdom with the best that science has to offer? Why do we feel ashamed of accessing what conventional medicine has to offer?

In the beginning, there was medicine. Medicine came from the earth, was largely the province of women, and mostly happened at home. Then came science, and medicine moved out of the home and primarily into the hands of men. Science is often ridiculed for being patriarchal and its value diminished—if not dismissed—in the name of intuition, innate wisdom, and healing. Medicine is often ridiculed, too, for similar reasons. It is time for the pendulum to swing toward the middle: there is so much to be gained from integrating science and intuition, and expert and individual experience.

## Functional Medicine Is Root-Cause Medicine

Functional medicine is root-cause medicine. It is the medicine of "why" as opposed to the medicine of "what." *Why* does someone feel a particular way as opposed to *what* disease they have and therefore which medication will make them feel

**Functional medicine is the medicine of "why"** as opposed to the medicine of "what."

———————————

better (obliterating, as opposed to resolving, their symptoms). Functional medicine identifies the root cause, and thus works toward the prevention and the treatment of complex, chronic disease. *Why* does she have fatigue? eczema? depression? She wasn't born that way. Something happened that changed her physiology.

Our health-care system is failing many of its patients. As a nation, we in the United States are sicker than we've ever been. According to the Centers for Disease Control, six in ten adults in our country have a chronic disease and four in ten adults have two or more. Chronic diseases and illnesses are largely the result of poor lifestyle choices. The trifecta of processed food, a sedentary lifestyle, and the majority of treatment for disease hinging on medication—or medications—is killing us. Crisis-care medicine has its time and place; thank goodness for surgery when we need it. However, crisis-care medicine is not designed to support or treat chronic conditions. We need a system for chronic conditions, and that system is functional medicine. We should not have to choose between crisis-care *and* functional medicine: ideally, everyone has access to both.

We are not solely to blame for our poor choices. The notion of "choice" is complex and influenced by socioeconomic status, education, geography, physical environment, employment, social support, and access. These variables are collectively referred to as the social determinants of health, and they have a huge impact on our health.

Let's not overlook the reality that being sick is big business, particularly for insurance and pharmaceutical companies. Discerning what is "healthy" is complicated by the amount of information or misinformation available on the internet, the bazillion-dollar health/self-help industry, and special-interest lobby groups affecting policy on everything from what constitutes standard of care to which foods provide which nutrients.

Discerning what is healthy requires varsity levels of sophistication. Then there is the challenge of navigating the health-care system—practitioners' offices, labs, hospitals, and insurance companies—largely oriented toward sickness as opposed to health.

The groundwork for functional medicine started in the 1950s, when progressive healers began to look at "natural" or "alternative" medicine. Discoveries about the nature of our bodies and the nutrients necessary to make them work were unfolding rapidly. Supplement companies began to form as a paradigm of treatment based on diet and nutritional therapies developed. Functional lab testing companies like Great Smokies Diagnostic Laboratory (now Genova Diagnostics) and Doctor's Data opened. During the 1980s, a small group of health-care professionals started to use nutrients, in the form of supplements and herbs, and lab-based data to determine treatments.

Among these health professionals was Dr. Jeffrey Bland, often referred to as the father of functional medicine. There were other fathers, as well, like doctors David Jones, Joe Pizzorno, and Mark Hyman. Dr. Bland coined the term "functional medicine" and started lecturing nationwide. Chiropractors, naturopaths, medical doctors, doctors of osteopathy, and acupuncturists started practicing functional medicine—lifestyle medicine based on laboratory testing with an emphasis on nutritional supplements and herbs.

Functional medicine grew in the 1990s as a system to treat chronic illnesses that were nonresponsive to conventional medicine. The Institute for Functional Medicine was founded in an effort to develop a formal training program and to move clinical medicine from the drug-based model of treating disease that worked well in the twentieth century to a systems-oriented, patient-focused clinical model designed to reduce the epidemic of chronic disease.

Systems biology is the science of wholeness and the science on which functional medicine is based. Our bodies contain a complex network of systems that interact with each other. Our organs exist within our physical bodies and, therefore, are subject to one another's influence. Everything, it turns out, is connected to everything.

Functional medicine practitioners consider the interconnections of an individual's history, physiology, genetics, and environment to answer the question, why? The practice considers internal factors, such as stress levels or what a person carries in her heart, and external factors, such as the quality of her community. Practicing functional medicine is about connecting seemingly unrelated symptoms. One cause can create many symptoms, and many causes can create one symptom. This is the medicine I practice, and I have done so for sixteen years.

There is so much we can do to take care of ourselves. Simple lifestyle interventions are game-changing when we know what they are and feel able to implement them. Changing our lifestyle is hard. *Really* hard. It might be the hardest thing we ever do. To change our lives without accurate information, without support, without a flat-out cheerleader, can feel daunting. Not to mention downright overwhelming. Most of us are overwhelmed most days. We frequently put others first. We struggle to give ourselves some of the time, money, and energy we extend toward others. The extent to which we care for others can significantly impact our own health—both positively and negatively.

## The Whole Picture

I have taken care of women for over twenty-four years. I spent the first part of my career practicing full-scope midwifery at my local community hospital, where I cared for women of all ages and stages, including during their childbearing years. The last birth I attended was in 2006. In August of that year, I started working at Women to Women, a pioneering women's health clinic that was located in Yarmouth, Maine.

When I got to Women to Women and started learning functional medicine, I could finally put words to all I had understood about health but had not had language for. I learned that auto-immune disease could present in children in their preteens; that it's ideal to teach young women about the importance of stress management and good nutrition so they are set up for a lifetime of hormone balance; and that a woman's first gyne-cologic exam can set the tone for her relationship with health care and health-care practitioners for life, so tread carefully. I discovered that caring for midlife women is remarkably similar to caring for a woman in labor—it's just a longer process with a slightly different outcome. The midlife transition does not *have* to be a crisis. When carefully tended, it results in the birth of a woman—beyond wife, mother, daughter, and whatever other roles she has. I learned that menopause is not a one-way train with a destination where we disembark. Menopause goes on for life. And that preventative measures, such as scheduling a mas-sage as part of routine maintenance as opposed to waiting until there is a problem, helps women age successfully. Functional medicine felt like—and continues to feel like—home, much the way midwifery does, even though I no longer tend births.

You don't have to wait until you're sick to take care of your-self. I want to help you see a whole picture, connect symptoms with root causes, transition to having health without a crisis, and be empowered to do what you can for yourself.

I WANT to make functional medicine accessible for *all* women. Functional medicine has a bit of a reputation for being elitist, available only to the affluent. It is true that food that comes

Functional medicine and a systems biology model **do not offer "pill for an ill" solutions.**

––––––––––––––––

from the earth typically costs more money than processed food, that functional tests are often not covered by health insurance companies, and that supplements are expensive. However, understanding the *why* of chronic disease and illness and the lifestyle interventions available to the masses is the intention of this book.

I hope to teach you that:

- what you eat profoundly affects your health

- seemingly unrelated symptoms are often connected, when looked at through a systems biology model

- the effect of stress on your health is not to be underestimated

- integrating intuition, lived experience, and science yields the best health care

- a medicine of *why* as opposed to a medicine of *what* can yield benefits for you and your family, for nations, and for the planet

This book is divided into two parts. In part one, "What Does It Mean to be Whole?" we'll explore concepts related to wholeness. We don't have to be perfect to be whole. We can be sick and whole simultaneously. We'll delve into the well-documented process of change so you can locate yourself within it and understand that change is not typically a linear process. I will introduce you to the Functional Medicine Matrix. We'll consider aspects of lifestyle that underwrite wholeness: without having your sleep, movement, nutrition, stress management, and relationships in order, it can be difficult to discern what your "real" health issues are. We'll also look at stress and trauma and how they affect our health. I present the concepts related to wholenesss first, for those readers who want a taste of the practical and theoretical underpinnings of functional medicine and my practice of it. This knowledge is meant to enrich your understanding of the second part of the book.

In part two, "The Nodes of the Matrix," I walk you through the seven core processes mapped out by functional medicine. They are the:

* Energy Node
* Communication Node
* Assimilation Node
* Biotransformation and Elimination Node
* Transport Node
* Defense and Repair Node
* Structural Integrity Node

Within each of the "node" chapters, I explain the node, introduce testing options that could reveal more about your health related to the node, and offer lifestyle, nutrition, and nutrient interventions. Functional medicine and a systems biology model do not offer "pill for an ill" solutions. No one thing on its own is likely to make you better. And addressing one nutrient or lifestyle modification within one node may reach far into another node as well. I share stories of women I have treated to illuminate common health concerns related to the nodes and a functional medicine approach to addressing them, which as you will see is rarely a straight path from point A to point B.

Those of you eager for tactical information may want to skip ahead and dive into those chapters in part two that call out to you. If you do, I encourage you to circle back to part one later for a richer understanding of how to apply the principles of functional medicine in your life.

## Walking Alongside You

While my work entails guiding women toward wholeness, know that I am right by your side. I, too, am a work in progress. I work on refining my lifestyle, asking myself, Can I do just a little bit better today? Some days the answer is yes, some days it is no, and some days it's simply, "I don't feel like it." I repeatedly cycle back to that which I "prescribe" to others, and, like you, I have wounds that I carry that affect how I walk through this world.

My hope is that this book serves as an introductory guide as you embark on a health-care journey that transcends conventional medicine. Nothing takes the place of expert guidance provided by a seasoned practitioner. I recommend that you seek to develop a health-care team—a team of practitioners you choose to help you care for yourself. Your team may include a medical doctor, a nurse practitioner, an acupuncturist, a therapist, a Rolfer, a nutritionist, a trainer... No one of us can do it all, nor do you have to go it alone.

There are some universalities to the female experience, yet each of our experiences is unique. Years of listening has resulted in a collective women's wisdom that warrants sharing. There is no finer comfort than knowing we are not alone in our experience. If this book can help you feel less alone, trust your intuition, look at your health in a more integrated way, find a team of skilled practitioners to support you, and inspire you to make changes for the better, I will have done my job.

# PART ONE

# what does it mean to be whole?

# 1

# Embracing
# the Mess

. . . . . . . . . . . . . . . . .

*INTEGRATING INTUITION AND
SCIENTIFIC WISDOM*

MANY WOMEN FEEL *as though they are at fault when they don't feel well. But you don't have to be perfect to be whole. You may not do everything you know would or could help yourself feel better, but beating yourself up about each and every transgression is a different kind of disease. Your "messes" or imperfections—the parts of yourself that make you human—are the realities within which to work as you move toward wholeness.*

FUNCTIONAL MEDICINE is the clinical practice of systems biology, or the science of wholeness. In this model, the body is considered a complex network of systems that interact with one another. Unlike the practice of conventional medicine, in which the body is treated as a fragmented collection of unrelated parts (if you have something wrong with your digestion, you see the gastroenterologist; your reproductive organs, a gynecologist; your hormones, the endocrinologist), systems biology unveils the complex interactions that happen within a biological system, such as the body, and aims to make sense of the interactions. Nothing in one part of the body is compartmentalized. All the parts are interrelated. The whole has greater potential for wellness than the sum of the parts. You are a whole woman.

And life is messy. We all have messes we manage—no one is exempt. Sometimes it takes courage to acknowledge the hard, challenging, imperfect parts of our lives. Sometimes the problems are so blatant that there is no looking away. You might be in a troubled relationship, have a life-threatening illness, or have acne no amount of makeup covers up.

The largest mess in my life occurred on June 8, 2018, when my daughter, Isabelle, died. Shortly after 5 p.m., I headed outside to greet friends who rolled into our driveway, to see if they wanted to share a gin and tonic. It was a warm, early summer evening and the last day of school for my husband who is a teacher, my friend, and my daughter. My son graduated from high school the weekend prior. He and I had spent the day mowing, weeding, and doing other outside chores. My husband was, of all things, repairing the snowblower in the garage. My daughter had been at a friend's house.

As I walked down the stone path to greet our friends, a sheriff's car was coming down our drive. The sheriff and his colleague parked, got out of their car, confirmed our names, and asked if we could go inside to talk. I was perplexed. What could they possibly want to talk to me about? What came next played out like a horror movie.

I sat on one of our two yellow couches in our sunroom, grungy and physically tired from a day of yardwork, the smell of fresh-mowed grass hanging in the air. The officer sat on our large, square, wooden coffee table, facing me, commenting on how difficult it is to sit with a bullet-proof vest on. He said, "There is no easy way to say this, but your daughter died in a car accident this afternoon."

Isabelle was fifteen years old when she passed. My daughter was healthy, kind, smart, and engaged. She loved ballet, skiing, sailing, her friends, and her family. I called her "My Lover of Life." She had recently gotten her driver's permit, had her first boyfriend of consequence who charmed her with an antique tin filled with homemade raspberry truffles, and she still had braces, which she was impatiently waiting to have removed.

Years of practice in positive thinking, visualization, and intention-setting blew up for me with Isabelle's passing. I used to end each of my journal-writing sessions with, "Please keep my children safe and well." If there is a god, or a higher power, or divination of any kind, I do not know or understand why my daughter died. Maybe she died for a reason, maybe it was her time, maybe sometimes shit just happens. I was close to the mysteries of life, tending births early in my career. Perhaps the only thing more mysterious than birth is death. I am now tethered to mystery forever.

We have some choice about how we meet the messes in our lives: we can either drown in them—the sickness, the infidelity, the uncertainty, the loss of whatever form—or we can alchemize them into a healing opportunity. Women respond to the death of their children, and other crises or tragedies, in a whole variety of ways, and I would guess that many don't feel like they have a choice about their response—it just is what it is. They

Messes, disorder, and crises
are moments rich with
**the potential for growing
and thus a gateway
to health and healing.**

———————

simply feel how they feel. I feel like I have a choice: I can wallow in all that is not and will never be, or I can take the deep loss I feel and redirect the intensity of that emotion into dancing, seeking or creating beauty, writing, or caring for others.

Messes, disorder, crises—these are the *crux* of life: moments rich with the potential for learning and growing and thus a gateway to health and healing. In the past, I was a rock climber and a rock-climbing teacher, which is when I was first introduced to the word "crux." The crux of a climb is the hardest move. At the crux of the climb, you either freak out because you are afraid, or your leg is shaking like you are pumping a sewing machine, or you are certain your forearms will explode. Back in the day, my freak-outs typically manifested as whimpering. Actually, they still do. When I am doing something physically challenging and I am afraid I can't do it or it feels too hard, I whimper. It's not my best look, but it happens—on the side of a mountain while skiing, on the hiking trail at the end of the day, on the stairs carrying something heavy and awkward to the attic. During the crux of a climb, though, a freak-out increases the likelihood of a fall. There is another choice: you can gather your mind, your breath, and your reason, and work it through. You learn a lot about yourself in those moments, and you get to practice your response.

Climbing is a phenomenal metaphor for the inevitable crux moments of life.

You can use the vulnerability you feel in the face of difficulty as an opportunity to get honest with yourself and make changes you previously thought unimaginable, or you can maintain your status quo.

Best-case scenario: you constantly assess and reassess your life, making micro-adjustments as you go—a little more exercise here, a new job there, more vegetables always. But rarely, in case you hadn't noticed, are the circumstances "best." In the business of life, most of us usually bumble along until there is a crisis—either delivered to our doorstep or of our own creation—and then we find ourselves on our knees, forced to grow. In twenty-plus years of clinical practice taking care of women, and in my own lived experience, I have observed that either we can voluntarily face the mess, or the mess will demand our attention often by manifesting as illness or disease. We are wise to face our messes willingly—and to elicit good counsel for help along the way.

## I Am You, You Are Me

Sometimes, as patients and clients, we do a funny thing to health-care practitioners: we elevate them above civilian status. The power differential created by thinking that someone else is better than us or has all the answers is reinforced by a patriarchal health-care system that historically purports the belief that "doctor knows best." A disassociation from our deep inner-knowing—that feeling that we know what is best for ourselves—disempowers us, increases the likelihood that we will regret our decisions, and contributes to medical trauma.

Your well-being depends on you being empowered to know, speak, and act on what is best for you.

Because of the untoward side effects of treatments that ultimately left them feeling no better, many women have regretted hysterectomies, invasive and extensive treatment for ductal carcinoma in situ, and hormone injections for pelvic pain that induced a medical menopause. I've heard too many women say, "If I knew then what I know now," or "I knew there were other ways. I just couldn't find someone to listen."

I sit in both chairs in my office—that of the patient and that of the practitioner. I do not know what treatment is best for someone else. I do not have health completely figured out—

mine or anyone else's. Nor am I perfect. I eat ice cream, fried clams, and birthday cake. I have challenging relationships. Sleep is a lifelong, ongoing challenge for me. I seek wholeness just like the women who come to see me. I learn as much from patients as I hope they learn from me.

Decades of collective women's wisdom, pattern observation, and clinical experience are what I bring to the practitioner-patient relationship. I see my job largely as being that of a tour guide: I discern what the root cause of a symptom might be and provide a continuum of options from which a woman can choose to begin healing. The woman's job is to identify what she is and isn't willing to do for the health she seeks. I am conscious of asking women to do that which would be difficult for me to do for the sake of health.

Humility, active listening, advocacy, and shared decision-making transform practitioner-patient relationships. Attention to these values results in patients feeling they have agency, or control, over their health journey. Agency begets a high level of accountability, resulting in a healthier lifestyle and the subsequent improved health. Together, patients and I review test results, consider treatment options, and make choices.

There is no way of knowing with certainty what an individual's experience of or outcome from an intervention is going to be. I can offer recommendations and guidelines based on research findings, but integrating each individual woman's experience into the decision-making process is crucial.

## You Weren't Born This Way

When I was a new, young registered nurse on the labor and delivery unit at Maine Medical Center, my mentor had been a nurse for as long as I'd been alive. She taught me this: listen to women. If the woman says the baby is coming, the baby is coming. Even if you just checked her and it seemed she had a long way to go. The last birth I attended was in 2006, but I still listen to women, and here's what I've learned: we generally have an intuitive sense of when and why our health went off the rails.

If you have a health condition and you *think* you know when it started and why, you are probably correct.

The vernacular is often the same: "I haven't been the same since..." I depend on women for the clues, if not the reveal, about what went wrong. The concern may be menopause, joint pain, diarrhea, constipation, autoimmune disease, acne, fatigue, heavy bleeding, or depression. To the women who don't know when or why, or when I'm challenged to identify the root cause of their concern, I say, "You weren't born this way. Something, or things, happened that tipped the balance in your body. Let's see if we can identify what happened."

Identifying *what happened* is one place where functional medicine and conventional medicine diverge. Medical diagnoses often reflect the patient's concern. They often go something like this:

Patient: "I can't leave the house because of frequent diarrhea."
Practitioner: "You have irritable bowel syndrome."

Labels are often limiting. I want to know *what happened to create the circumstances* resulting in an imbalance. How did the imbalance come to be? The heart of functional medicine is getting to the root cause of a symptom. *Why* do you have diarrhea? Not, *what* am I going to give you to make it stop?

Identifying antecedents, triggers, and mediators is part of the detective work:

* **antecedents** are predisposing genetic and environmental factors that someone brings to the table (the patient grew up near a paper mill)

- **triggers** are what activated the symptom (when estrogen drops before the patient's period, she gets a headache)

- **mediators** make symptoms better or worse (more than one glass of wine in the evening is a mediator that disrupts a patient's sleep)

When considering the "why" for a particular symptom or disease, it is important to remember that our genes are not our destiny. Just because we have a family history of high cholesterol does not mean we are doomed and destined to have high cholesterol. Genes are influenced by our environment, which leads to the expression of a gene. This field of study is referred to as epigenetics. When searching for the root cause of any health issue, consider how you live, think, and eat, your genes, and *all* the variables that influence your capacity for wellness and disease.

## What Do You Want Your Health For?

Women typically want to get well, be well, or stay well, for a reason. We want to leave the house without having to wear a diaper in fear of having an "accident." We want to be able to play on the floor with our grandchildren. We want to be able to get through a work meeting without feeling embarrassed by our soaking-wet blouse. Identifying the reasons we want to be well motivates us to change.

Women who come to see me are generally ready to change. Readiness for change is not to be taken for granted. It takes a lot to get ready. Getting ready is the necessary step before taking action.

Readiness may be cognitive, motivated by intellect, reason, and the mind, as in "I want to lower my blood pressure so I don't have a stroke." When the desire to change wells up from within, changes are better sustained. Women generally know what they need or want to do to take care of themselves, but the *doing* poses a challenge. Seeking support while you modify your lifestyle helps you implement the doing. This is midwifery care at its best—supporting women through education, love, and empowerment while they do hard things.

The process of change has been studied thoroughly and is broken into six phases.

1   **Precontemplation:** In this stage, people do not intend to act in the foreseeable future (defined as within the next six months). People are often unaware that their behavior is problematic or produces negative consequences. They often underestimate the pros of changing behavior and place too much emphasis on the cons of changing behavior. *A woman comes to the clinic and reports drinking five liters of diet soda a day (for real) and having debilitating muscle pain, unaware that diet soda may be the source of the problem. When educated about the possible connection, she finds the idea of not drinking diet soda unimaginable.*

2   **Contemplation:** In this stage, people intend to start a healthy behavior in the foreseeable future (defined as within the next six months). People recognize that their behavior may be problematic, and a more thoughtful and practical consideration of the pros and cons of changing the behavior takes place, with equal emphasis placed on both. Even with this recognition, people may still feel ambivalent about changing their behavior. *A perimenopausal woman has difficulty sleeping and knows her sleep is worse when she drinks wine in the evening; but still, she drinks it. She is in the contemplation stage of change.*

3   **Preparation (determination):** In this stage, people are ready to act within the next thirty days. They take small steps

Our genes
are not
**our destiny.**

———————

toward the behavior change, and they believe changing their behavior can lead to a healthier life. Sometimes test results serve as motivation, as does being "tired of feeling tired." At some point, lifestyle change seems easier than continuing to live with a symptom. *A woman with high blood pressure who has agreed to start exercising twice a week for thirty-minute sessions, with a plan to increase to five thirty-minute sessions a week within three months, is in the preparation stage of change.*

4   **Action:** In this stage, people have recently (within the last six months) changed their behavior and intend to maintain that change. People may exhibit this by modifying their problem behavior or acquiring new healthy behaviors. *A woman eats too many carbohydrates, feels sluggish, and subsequently does not want to exercise. Once she reduces her carbohydrate intake, she feels less sluggish and has improved energy and more motivation to exercise. More exercise improves her stamina, strength, and endurance, which begets regular exercise, which begets improved stamina, strength, and endurance, and so on.*

5   **Maintenance:** In this stage, people have sustained their behavior change for a while (for longer than six months) and intend to maintain the behavior change going forward. People in this stage work to prevent relapse to earlier stages. *A woman with a family history of alcoholism and a personal history of candida knows that when she eats cookies, "it's not one cookie, it is the whole box of cookies." After being treated for candida, she decides to not reintroduce processed sugar into her diet.*

6   **Termination:** In this stage, people have no desire to return to their unhealthy behaviors and are sure they will not relapse.

People rarely reach this point and tend to stay in the maintenance stage. *A woman says, "I'm never eating gluten again. It's just not worth it."*

I meet women wherever they are. I encourage you, too, to meet yourself wherever you are on the spectrum of change for whatever concern you are facing, because wherever you are is implicitly okay. Forcing yourself to be somewhere you are not is doing a disservice to yourself. You are on your own journey, influenced by too many variables to name, and possibly the only thing that matters at all is that you accept yourself exactly where you are.

We tend to have a difficult time being gentle with ourselves as we work toward change. Too often, when women come to the clinic for follow-up and "confess" they didn't follow the plan "perfectly," they say, "I was bad," or "I cheated." My heart breaks when I hear this self-deprecating language. Health-care practitioners are known to reinforce this kind of shame with language like "noncompliance," or "failed to . . ." But change is often two steps forward, one step back. It's generally not linear, and being hard on yourself makes it even more difficult to move forward.

I give you permission (if permission is needed) to be perfectly imperfect—otherwise known as *being human*—while you improve your health. You will benefit from putting yourself on the receiving end of the tender love you give to those around you when they embark on a challenging endeavor.

Determine what you are willing and not willing to do, for you. In *Mary Magdalene Revealed,* Meggan Watterson explains that for a woman to be able to change her life, she must feel agency. Without agency, you are simply following someone else's idea of what is good for you. The ethos of "doctor knows best" that permeates conventional medicine and protocol-based care annihilates agency, which is why conventional care so often fails. Listen to the quiet voice within you, the voice that comes in stillness and silence, the voice of knowing, down deep, what you want and why you want it for yourself.

## Be Your Own Health Expert

I have a vision in my head of what I look like in my best health. Maybe you have a vision too. And maybe also like me, your reality falls short of your vision. When push comes to shove, I have yet to be willing to do some of what I suspect might lead to my best health.

For example, I have never in my life been compelled to not eat cookies. I cannot imagine what circumstances would have to occur such that I would be motivated to cease the eating of cookies. I'm particular about the cookies I eat, but I still eat them. In general, I don't buy cookies from the grocery store. If I want a cookie, I make them (most of the time). I'm so happy when someone else makes cookies and gifts them to me so I can eat them without having to make them myself. Rarely, I will buy a cookie at a small bakery where things are made from scratch. For me, cookies are a small joy. I know my health would be better if I consumed less sugar and carbohydrates, and I find joy in other small things—but I also find joy in cookies. Joy is its own medicine. I believe that's true and not just an excuse to continue eating cookies.

Here's another example: I am unwilling to wake up at four in the morning to exercise. I have genuine, tremendous admiration for the women who do get up at 4 a.m., or whenever they have to get up before kids or work or whatever, to exercise. I just have never been compelled to do that. The circumstances under which I might be compelled to wake up at 4 a.m. to exercise are unimaginable to me. I've risen in the middle of the night to climb big mountains, on rare occasions. Waking in the dark to be active is not my norm.

Is it possible my health is limited by my choices? Absolutely. Less sugar and more exercise would certainly do me well. Like me, you probably have things you are willing and things you are unwilling to do for your health. Patients frequently draw a line in the sand when I suggest giving up coffee or wine. I'm generally glad when I encounter their resistance. Because being "perfect," or "doing everything right" is no insurance that your health remains intact. Too much rigidness and an uber-disciplined life can be detrimental to your health. There is no way to measure this, but you know it when you feel it. It might feel like:

- social isolation from not attending a gathering because you are following a restrictive diet

- impatience with your children because they interrupted your exercise schedule

- stress related to health-care costs from seeing many practitioners and trying many treatments in the spirit of getting healthy

Be honest with yourself about what you are willing to do for your health. Draw your lines where you want or need to. Use your intuition to guide your decision-making, but use science and the input from a seasoned practitioner as well. Ultimately, you are the expert of you.

## Finding Voice

When you engage with the conventional health-care system, it can be extraordinarily difficult to know where you stand within it. We engage because we are seeking help. We seek help

# Genes

# +

# environment

# =

# **expression**

---

because we don't feel well. Seeking help and not feeling well make us feel vulnerable. Feeling vulnerable makes it difficult to think and communicate clearly.

What follows is some of what I've learned from listening to women and from my own life experience about finding voice, confidence, and speaking up.

**It is difficult to find your voice if you don't make time, or have time, to connect with yourself.** When I worked full-time, was on call, and had two young children, there was little time for reflection. How was I to hear my own voice among the howls of laboring women at work and of toddlers at home? Eventually, the kids got older and more independent, and I got honest with myself about what I needed to be a sane human. I was able to identify that one of the things I needed was a bit of time alone. In silence and in solitude, I was able to discern my own voice. If you can, create even small windows of space and time where you need pay attention only to you.

**You need a corner of life where you can put down the mask that allegedly makes everything look okay.** Not only do you need a break from wearing your literal masks, but you need a break from your metaphorical masks too. You need a place where you can get real and quiet with yourself so you can hear the whisper of knowing that comes from within. The knowing that comes from within is your voice. The corner may be in the car commuting, in the bath, in the woods, in a place of worship, in the studio, or at the gym. Where the corner is matters not. What does matter is that you take off the mask you present to the world and dig beneath your surfaces to reveal and listen to the quiet, or perhaps raging, voice that lies underneath.

**You must talk yourself into believing you are enough.** My old colleague and dear friend Cate Gaynor, NP, taught me this mantra: "I am enough. I have enough. I do enough." I don't know the origins of this saying, but I know most of us feel like we "should" be doing more: Eating better. Drinking less. Exercising more. Advancing at work. Caring for our families. Making home. The incessant drive to do more will be the end of us, honestly. I cannot tell you the number of women I take care of who end up sick trying to do more than is possible because they think they can, life demands it, or they have difficulty saying no. Women's worthiness is dismissed in so many ways socially and culturally—for one example, according to the Pew Research Center, women earned 84 percent of what men earned at work in 2020. It's no wonder we have some unpacking to do around our sense of worth.

**No one is going to roll out a red carpet so you can take care of yourself.** You must believe you are worth some of the time, money, and energy you generously give to others and then bestow some of these resources upon yourself. It is unlikely anyone else can care for you in the deeply nourishing way you desire. Even those of us who have great moms or partners still have to mother ourselves. Practicing caring for yourself builds confidence that you can meet your own needs.

**When you do find your voice, people won't necessarily want to hear it.** Family members, employers, and co-workers become quite comfortable with us women doing more for others than we do for ourselves. You may worry that advocating for yourself in the health-care system will estrange you from the very people you hope will help you. You may be judged impractical or dismissed entirely. The best health-care plans are created when practitioners solicit women's involvement in the decision-making.

Voice means speaking, either to yourself or others, what you know to be true for you. I often hear women say, "I know there has to be a reason why," or "I don't want to take medication," or "I know this relationship is a barrier to my health." Finding voice, having voice, and using voice ensures you have a say in what is good for you, which is ultimately up to you to determine.

## Choice Is Crucial

As important as it is to find voice and to be honest with yourself, it is equally important to work with a practitioner who listens to you and meets you where you are. It's a waste of everyone's time to work with someone who doesn't hear you and asks you to do things you are unwilling or unable to do, financially or otherwise.

Penny is a mother of three who came to the clinic years ago with eczema, fatigue, and symptoms of menopause. She'd had a long history of skin rashes that started when her child's life was threatened. Because of Penny's personal trauma history, the threat to her child triggered a physiologic chain of events in her body.

Penny grew up in a home where she was emotionally abused by her parents. She had no recollection of sexual abuse, but she was unable to remember much of her childhood. She did remember the neglect she experienced.

After years of working together on her gut health, Penny told me she was experiencing pelvic pain. She hadn't had a pelvic exam for over a decade. She was terrified. I offered to order a pelvic ultrasound for her instead. But I also explained that best care involved a hands-on exam. There was information we could get from an exam that an ultrasound would not provide. Penny chose to have a pelvic exam.

Choice is crucial to empowerment. You can't be your own health expert if you don't know what possibilities exist and if no one is willing to teach you. Being educated about possibilities, discussing the risks and benefits of options, enables you to choose from a place of knowing. Participating in and having control over the decisions around your health care, as opposed to being told what to do, is an entirely different framework from what has historically been "power-over medicine." Choice increases empowerment and buy-in, ultimately resulting in better health.

2

# The Foundations of How You Live

· · · · · · · · · · · · · · · · · ·

*MODIFIABLE PERSONAL
LIFESTYLE FACTORS*

CONSIDERING AND ADDRESSING *personal lifestyle factors that you may have some control over—sleep, relaxation, exercise, nutrition, stress, and relationships—is the heart and soul of functional medicine. You may already know how you might modify your lifestyle to improve your health. Maybe it's going to bed earlier, maybe it's drinking less wine, maybe it's moving more. These changes can be the challenge of a lifetime! But health and wellness are not sustainable without a healthy lifestyle. How you live matters.*

EVERY CASE study in this book reveals a woman making different choices about the way she lives in order to feel better, whether she eliminates artificial sweeteners, exercises regularly, or works on unresolved emotional issues. Your health requires work only you can do for you. Aging requires we work even harder to maintain, or regain, health. This work does not come in the form of a pill. Sometimes, women with exquisite lifestyle choices still feel unwell. This can be particularly frustrating for both women and practitioners. A patient might feel frustrated, thinking, "I'm doing everything right, so why do I still feel so crummy?" When a patient's lifestyle choices are in order and she still feels unwell, a high level of clinical expertise is necessary to identify the root cause of the issue.

We make choices that collectively create our lifestyle and largely determine our health. These modifiable personal lifestyle factors include sleep and relaxation, exercise and movement, nutrition, stress, and relationships, and they influence every system in our bodies. Many health issues are resolved solely by making different lifestyle choices.

But resolving health issues can still be complex. Let's consider the example of true and false anxiety, as framed by Dr. Ellen Vora in her book, *The Anatomy of Anxiety*. False anxiety is no less real than true anxiety in its felt experience. But false anxiety is a response to a physiologic process such as increased cortisol (the fight-or-flight hormone produced by the adrenal glands) during a stressful time or erratic blood sugar from skipping meals. So for some people, anxiety can be remedied by managing stress, decreasing cortisol levels, and regularly eating food that stabilizes blood sugar. After cortisol and blood sugar issues are addressed, then true anxiety can be dealt with, whether its roots are in trauma, identity, or purpose. Dr. Vora talks about using true anxiety as a North Star, an indicator that something—a job, a relationship, a social engagement—is "not quite right" here.

Such as it is with every diagnosis or health issue: The symptom is the end of the road, not the beginning. Is there something at the beginning of the road that can be addressed so the end of the road is never reached? Addressing modifiable lifestyle factors may be just the thing.

## Stress

Stress affects our health in *every* way: blood pressure, sleep, blood sugar regulation, thought processes, breathing, muscle tension, and metabolism, to name a few. Our culture rewards high stress. We wear it like a badge of honor. When stress levels are high, it is *incredibly challenging* to be well. I met with a nurse who works in the emergency room at a city hospital where many people with mental illness go. She told me the story of caring for a patient with schizophrenia who arrived at the emergency room with self-inflicted cuts bleeding down her arms. The nurse, following protocol, accompanied the patient into a locked room while the patient changed, having to trust the patient's word that the razor blade with which she cut herself was in a bag outside the changing room. The nurse recalled the stress of that encounter and how it tapped into her own trauma. At the end of her visit with me, this nurse, my patient, asked me why she might be sleeping for ten hours a day. I explained the physiology of stress and the cumulative effect of it on her sleep-wake cycle. Sleep is one way the body tries to recover from secreting large amounts of cortisol when experiencing stress. Fortunately, the nurse has a new job. Eliminating the stress of working in an emergency room will enable her to restore her health more expeditiously than if she regularly continued to be in such a high-stress environment.

## Relationships
. . . . . . . . . . . . . . . .

The number and strength of our relationships affect our well-being. An emerging field of science called sociogenomics studies how relationships influence the expression of our genes. Healthy relationships are associated with lower incidences of anxiety and depression, higher self-esteem, a strong immune system, and even a longer life.

Loneliness can lead to poor sleep, high blood pressure, or an increase in cortisol levels. Loneliness is also correlated with increased incidences of obesity and inflammation, and is a precursor to heart disease, stroke, and cancer. The COVID-19 pandemic shined a light on how relationships affect our health. There were increased incidences of teen anxiety and depression during the pandemic, largely the result of isolating, quarantining, and at-home school.

If you feel a dearth of healthy relationships in your life, think creatively about how you might foster them. Maybe it's through a hiking club or book group, or by volunteering at a local food bank. Let your curiosities and interests direct where you put your attention. Sharing a common interest with someone can provide a rich foundation to a new relationship. If you are content with the relationships in your life, send a note of gratitude to those folks with whom you share them for the roles they play in your life.

## Exercise and Movement
. . . . . . . . . . . . . . . . . . . . . . . . . .

No single pill improves our health as much as routine exercise and movement. The benefits of exercise are too great in number to fully list, but here are a few. Exercise decreases stress levels and improves:

- blood pressure
- heart health
- strength and mobility
- hormone balance
- digestion

Incorporating exercise and movement into your lifestyle isn't a matter of *having* time, it's a matter of *making* time. For some of us, it has to be a stake in the ground around which the other parts of life happen. One of my primary strategies to incorporate exercise into my life when my kids were little was to exercise *with* them. We had a jogger I could take to the local nature preserve and push them in while walking or jogging; I carried them in a backpack while hiking and skiing; we invested in child-sized gardening tools so they could join us in the yardwork. Incorporating yoga into my lifestyle was a challenge until I found a kid's yoga video they enjoyed and I could simultaneously do my own stretching. When they got older and had ski racing practice, I would ski, too, or walk with the dog. When I drove Isabelle to dance, sometimes I would go for a walk or a run on the bike path while she was at class.

Sharing exercise and movement with my children resulted in a family culture of spending time outdoors being active. To this day, some of the best time we spend together is skiing or walking. I'm beyond grateful for their love of all things outdoors, and for what was Isabelle's love of dance. Their active lifestyle provided them a healthy outlet for coping with the stressors of growing up.

There are numerous strategies to try as you work exercise and movement into your lifestyle: Paying for a gym membership or a trainer helps some women maintain accountability. Other women benefit from consistently exercising with a friend. Some women enjoy the social aspect of group classes. If you are sedentary, start with a walk around the block at the end of the workday as a way to transition from work to home. Over time, you can build on that small success by lengthening the time, frequency, or intensity of the walk, as well as incorporating other types of exercise.

## Nutrition

Most of us have tremendous agency over what we put on the end of our fork and into our mouth. Food is our first medicine. Junk in, junk out. Eating food that we could hunt or gather is the food that is best for us. In its absence, a multitude of health issues can arise. In its presence, a multitude of health issues resolve.

### FOUNDATION SUPPLEMENTS

The following are supplements I recommend to enhance health in each node of the matrix and for health maintenance when we are well:

- **Multivitamins:** Help ensure basic nutrient requirements are met in case you are not getting them through your food. Think of taking a multivitamin like putting toner in a copy machine.

- **Vitamin D3:** Functions more like a hormone than a vitamin. Vitamin D3 is essential for mood support, immune system support, and bone health.

- **Omega-3 fatty acids:** Good for eyes, hair, skin, and nails, as well as neurologic function and immune system protection. Omega-3s have far-reaching anti-inflammatory effects.

No single pill improves
our health as much
as **regular exercise
and movement.**

---

- **Probiotics:** Help ensure we have adequate good bacteria in our guts. Rotate between at least three different products. Each product has specific organisms, and you want to get a cross-section of organisms.

Women over fifty can consider adding:

- **B complex:** Essential for many physiologic processes. B vitamins support mood and energy.

- **CoQ10:** A potent antioxidant that declines in us with age.

## Relaxation

You probably have a lot to do, almost always. At least that's how it is in my world and in those of many of my patients too. Like exercise, relaxation is something most of us have to *make* time for. We have to choose it—let the chores go unfinished, the house go uncleaned, the extra work for our jobs go undone. Some might say it's a privileged choice, and I see that. For those of us with the privilege, the choice can still feel difficult.

The health benefits of relaxation are extensive—decreased incidences of depression, decreased blood pressure, improved sleep, improved digestion, and decreased inflammation, to name a few. This is lifestyle medicine.

## How You Live Matters

Incorporating personal lifestyle modifications into a plan of care—supporting someone as they make different choices about the way they live—is one of the most significant factors differentiating functional medicine from conventional medicine.

In functional medicine, restoring health is not solely dependent upon whether or not someone took their medication. Nor does a person's health lay solely in the hands of the practitioner. It is not entirely up to me to "make" someone better any more than it is up to someone else to help me feel better. If I tear a ligament in my knee and I want to continue to hike and ski, I put my health in the hands of the surgeon for the surgery. But after surgery, a full recovery depends on my participation in physical therapy. Similarly, if I'm in a major motor vehicle accident and I'm bleeding internally, I am grateful to the surgeon who can stop the bleeding. In those scenarios, I completely hand over my power to the practitioner. But only temporarily.

Now, if I have high blood pressure and a family history of high blood pressure, and I am not exercising regularly or eating lots of vegetables, and I do not have a spiritual practice that quiets my central nervous system, why would I, or my healthcare practitioner, expect a pill to correct my blood pressure—especially given the frequent ineffectiveness of blood pressure medication? When one medication fails to treat high blood pressure, a second medication is often prescribed. Even when medication normalizes blood pressure, the underlying biochemical imbalance causing the high blood pressure will manifest as another symptom in another system.

Conventional medicine treats symptoms. Conventional medical practitioners typically prescribe a "pill for an ill." Taking multiple medications, also known as polypharmacy, creates its own health problems. The net effect of any particular cocktail of medications is unstudied, thereby making it impossible to distinguish symptoms from what might be the cumulative effects of taking multiple medications. When the line between what is a symptom and what are the cumulative side effects of medical treatment of a symptom becomes murky, the importance of getting to the root cause is even more important.

Addressing modifiable lifestyle factors is about doing what we can to have the health we seek. It's about tabling the false expectation that something or someone can or will make you better. Other things and people can help, for sure. But for optimal health, your participation is required.

# 3

# Making Sense of Your Symptoms

. . . . . . . . . . . . . . . . . . . .

*THE TOOLS OF
FUNCTIONAL MEDICINE*

SYMPTOMS ARE EXPRESSIONS *of physiologic imbalances. Symptoms are not, in and of themselves, the problem. The problem is in the change in physiology that creates symptoms. Functional medicine practitioners aim to correct underlying physiologic imbalances, which is why functional medicine is referred to as root-cause medicine. Ideally, when physiology is rebalanced, symptoms resolve. Seemingly unrelated symptoms may share an underlying physiologic imbalance, and because everything is connected to everything, correcting one imbalance can improve a variety of symptoms. You are a complex web of interactions.*

THE FOCUS in functional medicine is on understanding the "why" of your symptoms. You were likely not born with whatever now troubles you. Something changed your biochemistry, that changed your physiology, that is now manifesting as a physical symptom. The "thing" that changes your biochemistry could be eating foods that were inflammatory for you as an infant, taking multiple rounds of antibiotics, trauma, international travel, hospitalization or surgery, any of the hormone shifts that happen in your life, or stress.

Functional medicine practitioners incorporate the interconnections of an individual's history, physiology, genetics, and environment to get at the root cause of an illness. Internal factors, such as the state of someone's spirit, and external factors, such as their social environment, are also considered. Functional medicine is like drawing a constellation, connecting individual dots to create a picture. Often, seemingly unrelated symptoms are connected by a common cause. There can be one cause for many symptoms, and there can be many causes for one symptom.

As a functional medicine practitioner, I focus on identifying the underlying mechanism, or root cause, of symptoms. I work to understand where the error in biochemistry is occurring. Which specific autoimmune disease someone has is less interesting to me than understanding what turned the immune system on and what keeps it going. Yes, immune systems get activated. Because typically, if someone has *one* autoimmune disease, they have *more than one*. If they don't have more than one autoimmune disease now, unless and until the root cause is resolved, the inflammatory cascade will continue to occur and move from system to system until it is stopped. The home of the immune system, and thus autoimmune disease, is primarily in the gut. When I address the gut, all autoimmune diseases are being addressed.

## One Condition, Many Imbalances

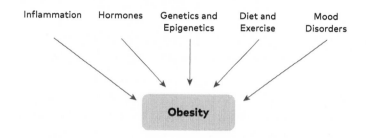

## One Imbalance, Many Conditions

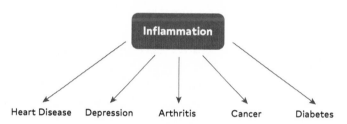

Functional medicine shifts the disease-centered focus of conventional medical practice to a client-centered approach. The whole person is considered, not just her isolated symptoms. Care is time-intensive and unique to each individual. Conventional medical practices are combined with integrative medical practices. Therapeutic nutritional interventions, lifestyle modifications, and exercise are primary interventions. Laboratory testing is used, some conventional, some functional. Supplements, herbs, or medications are also used as needed, depending on the circumstances and individual preference. Treating people as individuals, or what is referred to as personalized medicine, is quite effective.

If you haven't gotten better through conventional medicine, or you know some of your symptoms are connected in a way your practitioner is not acknowledging, or you want to know what you can do other than take medication for a particular issue, functional medicine may be for you.

The Institute for Functional Medicine has multiple teaching tools that help practitioners organize symptoms and data to identify the root causes of a person's imbalances. This is necessary in a systems model, where everything is connected to everything. No one system exists in isolation. Systems exist within the context of the whole person and, for that matter, the universe. As physical beings, we interact with life on Earth as well as with that which we cannot see. Quantum physics is the field of science revealing the interconnectedness of living material and non-material systems. The mystery contained within us, and around us, still transcends scientific explanation. We do not yet, and may not ever, fully understand the body, or life, or why what happens happens. Though it makes many conventional practitioners quite uncomfortable, I find solace in the magic and mystery of life, and I will delve further into interconnectedness in the pages to come.

The three primary tools used by functional medicine practitioners are the Functional Medicine Matrix, the Functional Medicine Timeline, and the Medical Symptom Questionnaire (MSQ).

## The Functional Medicine Matrix

The matrix offers a structure by which to organize symptoms. Through using the matrix, a visual concentration of imbalances in individual biological systems, called nodes, emerges:

- The **Energy Node** relates to how the body makes energy on the cellular level.

**"I've never been the same since..."** is the language of a woman telling me what activated, or which event triggered, the onset of her symptoms.

———————————

- The **Communication Node** relates to hormones, neurotransmitters, immune messaging, and how the body sends messages between systems.

- The **Assimilation Node** relates to digestion and our microbiome, the organisms living within the digestive tract.

- The **Biotransformation and Elimination Node** relates to how the body transforms nutrients and eliminates toxins.

- The **Transport Node** relates to the cardiovascular and lymphatic systems.

- The **Defense and Repair Node** relates to the immune system, infection, and inflammation.

- The **Structural Integrity Node** relates to the integrity of cells, like the ones that make up the arteries and veins, and the musculoskeletal system.

Like a spider web when one thread is pulled and the shape of the web changes, such it is, too, with working the matrix. When you affect one node, the other nodes are affected as well.

At the center of the matrix are three interrelated health factors: mental, emotional, and spiritual. Mental health refers to cognitive function and perceptual patterns. Emotional health refers to emotional regulation, grief, sadness, anger, et cetera. Spiritual health refers to our sense of meaning and purpose, as well as our relationship with something greater. These three factors of health underwrite our entire physiology. We'll dive a little deeper into these factors in the next chapter.

Included in the matrix are the categories of antecedents, triggers, and mediators we talked about in chapter 1. Antecedents are the predisposing factors, including genetic and environmental factors; triggering events, meaning activators, are what started the problem; and mediators, or perpetuators, are what mitigate, or perpetuate, the symptoms. This aspect of the matrix captures the patient's story, which may go something like, "I had lots of ear infections [antecedent] when I was an infant, then I had recurrent strep throat [triggering event] in my teens. In my twenties I suffered from recurrent urinary tract infections [triggering event], and now, when I eat dairy [mediator/perpetuator], I have diarrhea."

When I consider antecedents, I look at things like the patient's environment when she was in utero. The study of epigenetics explores the impact of the external environment on developing embryos and the subsequent health implications. While I consider genetic predisposition, like a family history of high blood pressure or celiac disease, our genes, as has been previously explained, do not fully determine our destinies. I also consider factors like chronic stress and geography. An island near my home is down-river from a nuclear power plant that has since closed. There is a high incidence of thyroid cancer within the small island community. It is possible that something from the nuclear power plant contaminates the air or water and predisposes individuals to thyroid cancer.

Recall that "I've never been the same since..." is the language of a woman telling me what activated, or which event triggered, the onset of her symptoms. Women are not always this clear, but when they are, my job feels easy! There has to be enough time for the woman to tell her story, and for me to listen to what she has to say, for us to identify her triggers. Triggers include things like significant loss or death, international travel, having a baby, an insect bite, or taking antibiotics.

Mediators and perpetuators can sound like:

- "I know when I'm running routinely, my menstrual cramps are not as bad."
- "I know if I drink two glasses of red wine, instead of one, I will not sleep well."
- "I feel better when I meditate daily."

Mediators and perpetuators are often lifestyle choices, the things we do that influence our health. When working to understand your health as it is, it may be helpful to think about what the environment that you grew up in was like (antecedents), what events happened in your life that may have contributed to you not feeling well (triggers), and what now makes you feel better or worse (mediators).

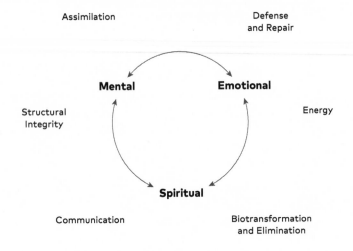

## Functional Medicine Matrix

### Physiology and Function:
### Organizing the Patient's Clinical Imbalances

Assimilation

Defense
and Repair

**Mental**

**Emotional**

Structural
Integrity

Energy

**Spiritual**

Communication

Biotransformation
and Elimination

Transport

## Retelling the Patient's Story

ANTECEDENTS

_____

_____

TRIGGERING EVENTS

_____

_____

MEDIATORS/PERPETUATORS

_____

_____

## Modifiable Personal Lifestyle Factors

SLEEP & RELAXATION

_____

_____

EXERCISE & MOVEMENT

_____

_____

NUTRITION

_____

_____

STRESS

_____

_____

RELATIONSHIPS

_____

_____

## The Functional Medicine Timeline

The Functional Medicine Timeline is a history-taking tool created by the Institute for Functional Medicine. The timeline is used to organize a patient's experience such that both clinician and patient better understand the causes of their illness. The timeline gives patients insight into their lives and validates that they have been heard. Perspective and validation motivate patients to make lifestyle modifications and engage in their health care.

Sometimes, women work on their timelines outside the clinic. It can be difficult to remember the exact sequence of events in our lives, especially when there are lots of details, like complicated surgical histories, visits with multiple practitioners, or trials of different medications. I took care of a woman who made her timeline an art project. She created a spiral on watercolor paper. She wrote in significant life events—births, deaths, moves, surgeries, and so on. Her process revealed influential events that affected her health. The art was a beautiful tribute to her life.

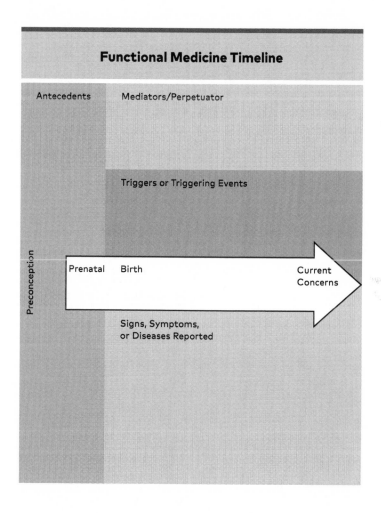

**Functional Medicine Timeline**

Antecedents

Mediators/Perpetuator

Triggers or Triggering Events

Preconception

Prenatal    Birth

Current
Concerns

Signs, Symptoms,
or Diseases Reported

We "work the nodes of the matrix" until a person is where they want to be with their health.

———————————

The timeline incorporates antecedents, triggering events, and mediators/perpetuators across the lifespan. Signs, symptoms, and diseases are reported. The timeline starts with preconception—often neglected is the health of a woman's mother when she was conceived, what life was like for her mom when she was in utero, and the details of her birth—and ends with current concerns.

I recommend that you spend some time charting out a timeline of your own health history and important events in your life to begin to piece together the story of your own health. You could use a structure like the timeline included or get creative like my client who made her timeline into an art piece.

## The Medical Symptoms Questionnaire

The Medical Symptoms Questionnaire (MSQ) is a third tool created by the Institute for Functional Medicine that I use to evaluate women's symptoms and monitor their progress. Patients complete this questionnaire prior to their first visit as part of their new-patient paperwork. A numeric value is assigned to a symptom, reflecting its severity. Symptoms are loosely clustered by nodes. The section with the highest score directs me toward which node likely has the strongest imbalance.

The MSQ is particularly helpful when a patient is not feeling better or does not seem to be improving. A patient can complete the questionnaire periodically so we can see when and if her health has changed. The MSQ provides a way to measure progress. Sometimes improvements come in baby steps, and it can be difficult to discern if there is any progress at all. If a treatment plan truly isn't working, it's on me to determine why and refine the plan. If a woman is willing to restrict her food choices for a period of time and spend a lot of money on supplements, I want to be sure she is getting better.

## Medical Symptoms Questionnaire (MSQ)

Patient Name _____

Date _____

Rate each of the following symptoms based on your typical health profile for the past two weeks using the following point scale:

0   Never or almost never have the symptom

1   Occasionally have the symptom, effect is not severe

2   Occasionally have the symptom, effect is severe

3   Frequently have the symptom, effect is not severe

4   Frequently have the symptom, effect is severe

**Head**

_____   Headaches

_____   Faintness

_____   Dizziness

_____   Insomnia                              _____ **TOTAL**

## Eyes

_____ Watery or itchy eyes

_____ Swollen, reddened, or sticky eyelids

_____ Bags or dark circles under eyes

_____ Blurred or tunnel vision (Does not
include near- or far-sightedness)    _____ **TOTAL**

## Ears

_____ Itchy ears

_____ Earaches, ear infections

_____ Drainage from ear

_____ Ringing in ears, hearing loss    _____ **TOTAL**

## Nose

_____ Stuffy nose

_____ Sinus problems

_____ Hay fever

_____ Sneezing attacks

_____ Excessive mucus formation    _____ **TOTAL**

## Mouth/Throat

_____ Chronic coughing

_____ Gagging, frequent need to clear throat

_____ Sore throat, hoarseness, loss of voice

_____ Swollen or discolored tongue, gums, lips

_____ Canker sores                    _____ **TOTAL**

## Skin

_____ Acne

_____ Hives, rashes, dry skin

_____ Hair loss

_____ Flushing, hot flashes

_____ Excessive sweating              _____ **TOTAL**

## Heart

_____ Irregular or skipped heartbeat

_____ Rapid or pounding heartbeat

_____ Chest pain                      _____ **TOTAL**

## Lungs

_____ Chest congestion

_____ Asthma, bronchitis

_____ Shortness of breath

_____ Difficulty breathing          _____ **TOTAL**

## Digestive Tract

_____ Nausea, vomiting

_____ Diarrhea

_____ Constipation

_____ Bloated feeling

_____ Belching, passing gas

_____ Heartburn

_____ Intestinal or stomach pain          _____ **TOTAL**

## Joints/Muscles

_____ Pain or aches in joints

_____ Arthritis

_____ Stiffness or limitation of movement

_____ Pain or aches in muscles

_____ Feeling of weakness or tiredness          _____ **TOTAL**

## Weight

_____ Binge eating or drinking

_____ Craving certain foods

_____ Excessive weight

_____ Compulsive eating

_____ Water retention

_____ Underweight                    _____ **TOTAL**

## Energy/Activity

_____ Fatigue, sluggishness

_____ Apathy, lethargy

_____ Hyperactivity

_____ Restlessness                    _____ **TOTAL**

## Emotions

_____ Mood swings

_____ Anxiety, fear, nervousness

_____ Anger, irritability, aggressiveness

_____ Depression                      _____ **TOTAL**

### Mind

_____ Poor memory

_____ Confusion, poor comprehension

_____ Poor concentration

_____ Poor physical coordination

_____ Difficulty in making decisions

_____ Stuttering or stammering

_____ Slurred speech

_____ Learning disabilities _____ **TOTAL**

### Other

_____ Frequent illness

_____ Frequent or urgent urination

_____ Genital itch or discharge _____ **TOTAL**

### Grand Total _____

A woman may present to the clinic with the primary concern of fatigue. Fatigue can have a variety of causes, stemming from a variety of nodes, for example:

- Not enough cortisol production is a Communication Node imbalance.

- Not enough iron in the blood is a Transport Node imbalance.

* Exposure to mold toxicity is a Biotransformation and Elimination Node imbalance.

Focusing attention on only one node often limits the extent to which people get well. In functional medicine, we "work the nodes of the matrix" until a person is where they want to be with their health. The tools are presented here to prompt a reconceptualization, and thereby a better understanding, of your health, one in which your mind, body, and spirit are integrated, your health journey has relevance, and your symptoms are the manifestations of physiologic imbalance.

# 4

# The Underwriters of Health

. . . . . . . . . . . . . . . . . . .

*THE CENTER OF THE MATRIX*

THE MIND, BODY, AND SPIRIT *are connected, affecting each other and every node of the Functional Medicine Matrix. These factors are the focal point of the matrix. Optimal health requires we address these factors. Unhealed trauma profoundly affects our physical and emotional health in a multitude of ways. Unhealed trauma may be a contributing factor to, or the root cause of, sexual dysfunction, disordered eating, insomnia, or addiction. Our physical health is intricately intertwined with mental, emotional, and spiritual factors.*

WE TOUCHED on the center of the matrix in the previous chapter. These three interlocking factors of mental, emotional, and spiritual health underwrite our entire physiology. Mental health refers to cognition and perceptual patterns. Emotional health refers to emotional regulation—how grief, sadness, anger, and so on are dealt with. Spiritual health refers to sense of purpose as well as a relationship with something greater.

## Mental Health

The Institute for Functional Medicine defines mental factors as elements related to cognitive function and perceptual patterns. Women commonly report "foggy thinking" as a primary symptom when they come to the clinic. I try to be mindful about how overwhelming a first visit can be in length and scope, about how confusing it can be to vet different testing options, about the financial impact of using tests often not covered or only partially covered by health insurance, and about a patient's capacity to make significant dietary changes or follow a complex supplement regimen.

### How you think affects your body

The biological pathways of your thoughts affect every cell in your body. Bruce Lipton outlines this process in his book *The Biology of Belief*. Is the cup half empty or half full? Is cancer a death sentence or an opportunity to shed the disingenuous parts of your life and live more earnestly? Does conventional medicine help or hinder? Do you approach health-care practitioners as your advocates or your adversaries? Do you feel like you have to "fight" for the care you want? Your thoughts and subsequent perceptions and their patterns have tremendous impact on your health and your decisions about it.

The science of gratitude elucidates this nicely. When you express or receive gratitude, your brain releases dopamine and serotonin, two "feel good" hormones. Not only do you *feel* happier but also your immune system is strengthened and you experience fewer or decreased body aches and pains, sleep better, and lower your blood pressure. According to studies on the neuroscience of positive thinking, gratitude also affords social benefits like better communication and stronger relationships.

Perceptions influence your decision-making around your health too. One woman with depression may want medication, certain it will help her feel better. A different woman may be open to trying anything *but* medication, certain the risks of medication outweigh the benefits. Some women think that it's impossible that what they eat affects their health, or that exercising despite feeling exhausted will result in more energy. Some think that having one bowel movement a week is normal.

Diagnoses like mild cognitive impairment or dementia impact women's health not only directly in terms of their ability to actually remember details but also in terms of how health-care services are delivered. Women with memory issues typically come to the clinic with a family member advocating on their behalf. I am grateful for the family member's presence in terms of helping both with history-taking and with the woman's processing of the visit later. But I am also wary when a woman does not speak for herself. I am curious: What would *she* say about her experience? What are her preferences? It requires skillful negotiation for three people to make a plan of care, especially when the patient's cognitive, or mental, capacity is compromised.

## Emotional Health

Emotional health refers to emotional regulation, grief, sadness, and anger. Therapeutic nutrition interventions are one of the most powerful treatments tools I use. I disdain the word "diet" and all the associated implications of "dieting." As previously stated, food is your first medicine, and as such, food can help or hinder your health. But even therapeutic nutrition interventions can trigger emotions for women—feelings of oppression, lack of control, or rebellion, to name a few.

I took care of a woman experiencing chronic constipation. We identified candida overgrowth as the source of the issue. I recommended an Anti-Candida Food Plan as part of her treatment. She struggled with this recommendation. She shared that when she was a teenager, she stopped eating in an effort to make her mother angry. That I was telling her what she could and could not eat triggered this childhood experience in her. She was unable to follow the food plan until she'd done some counseling and worked through her history around food and her mother.

Emotional regulation, or untended dysregulation, can obstruct your path to wellness. Sometimes a woman does not get better, despite our best efforts, both hers and mine. When all possible physiologic imbalances have been addressed and someone still does not feel better, I consider the possibility that trauma and the resultant dysregulated nervous system are undermining her health.

According to expert Irene Lyon, unhealed trauma may be the root cause of disease when a woman:

- is resistant to change
- procrastinates or is unable to move her life forward
- is unwell despite significant dietary modifications

Stress can change **the shape of the brain.**

---

- experiences anxiety and fear for no reason
- has a pattern of toxic relationships and self-sabotage
- has chronic health conditions

## Trauma

Trauma occurs when the physical feelings of a stressful experience persist in the body beyond the actual event. In *The Myth of Normal*, Dr. Gabor Maté differentiates "big T trauma" from "little T trauma." Big T traumas are such traumatic events as abuse of any kind, proximity to war, or a plane crash. Little T traumas are what occur to us on a personal level, like the loss of a pet. Maté further explains that trauma is less about what actually happened and more about our *experience* of what happened.

Stressful experiences—traumas of any shape or size—can change the physical structure of the brain.

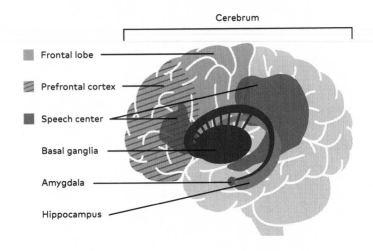

Let that sink in. Stress can change the shape of the brain.

When structure changes, function changes. The structure and function of the amygdala, hippocampus, and prefrontal cortex can change in response to stress. Trauma can cause a person to respond to subsequent stressors with increased cortisol and norepinephrine such that the response may be disproportionate to the situation.

Most of us have experienced trauma in our lives—a car accident, divorce, bullying, abortion, war, gun violence, rape or assault, birth, physical abuse, tragic death, systemic racism, and workplace discrimination are just a few examples. Irene Lyon identifies four types of trauma:

1   **Shock:** The result of an accident, broken limb, natural disaster, or abuse.

2   **Accumulated stress:** The cumulative effect of industrialized living, working too much, and not having enough unstructured time.

3   **Medical:** The result of medical treatment or encounters with health-care practitioners or the health-care system, anesthesia, near-death experiences, or poor treatment.

4   **Early and developmental trauma:** The result of bad and scary things that happen under the age of three, as well as in-utero stress, birth trauma, prematurity, health scares, and surgery.

Trauma activates our survival mechanisms of fight, flight, and freeze. Our survival mechanisms are driven by the part of the central nervous system (CNS) called the autonomic nervous system (ANS), or the automatic part of our nervous system. The ANS controls things like heart rate, blood pressure, digestion, and the immune system. When the ANS is chronically activated, all body systems suffer. Ideally, the ANS triggers the sympathetic nervous system (SNS), which puts a person into action.

During trauma, the lateral amygdala is activated. The amygdala is the smoke detector of the brain that sends out warning signals that things are not right. The message then travels to the basal ganglia, the part of the brain that controls movement. If we can *do* something about the threat we are experiencing, like fight back or run away, the stress cycle ends.

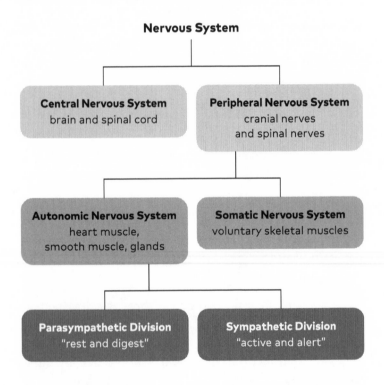

When action is not possible, the ANS remains activated. When we cannot act, the basal ganglia sends messages to the center of the amygdala, imprints a cycle of pain and fear, and stimulates a cycle of stress hormone production. We do irrational things when we operate from the survival center of the brain because the rational brain has no access to the emotional brain. This is the mechanism by which trauma ingrains itself in our physiology. Healing trauma requires healing our brains and our nervous systems.

Additionally, the frontal lobe of our brain *stops working* when we experience trauma. The frontal lobe is responsible for thinking and reasoning. We don't think clearly or reasonably when we are experiencing trauma. Our speech center (for most people, the left side of the cerebrum) stops working, too, which makes healing from trauma even more difficult. Talking about trauma may be impossible or retraumatizing for survivors.

Dr. Stephen Porges developed the polyvagal theory, which advances our understanding of ANS reactivity beyond the fight-or-flight response, expanding it to include freezing or immobilization. Freezing is when we feign death, pass out, or shut down in response to an unsafe situation. Polyvagal theory proposes that our central nervous system is constantly evaluating our environment for safety or danger. We get that information not just through perception but also through neuroception. Neuroception is the subconscious way the body processes information about the environment. A person's response to these cues is involuntary, like a baby cooing at a caregiver and crying with a stranger. The nervous system of someone in a constantly dangerous environment can have difficulty detecting safety. Thus, the individual tends to be reactive and is prone to misreading people's cues. You likely know someone for whom this is true or can imagine the havoc this wreaks in interpersonal relationships. You may even see this in yourself.

In 1985, Dr. Vincent Felitti conducted a weight-loss study in San Diego. He observed that people who lost weight dropped out of the study. Further investigation revealed that people who did not lose weight and stayed in the study had experienced abuse, often sexual abuse, often by a family member. He coined these traumatic experiences "adverse childhood events" (ACEs). The ACEs study correlated early childhood stress and adversity with people having an increased risk of cancer, heart disease, chronic illness, mental illness, being victims of violence, and having violent tendencies.

Healing trauma requires healing **our brains, our nervous systems, and our guts.**

———————

Talking about trauma for trauma survivors often activates their symptoms. Meditation and mindfulness practices can be excruciating for them. Healing trauma involves teaching the body it is safe. This is accomplished by mastering stress physiology through a body-based approach, not through the brain.

We can teach the body it is safe by building regulation. We build regulation through restoring physiologic function and changing neurological pathways in the brain. Furthermore, Dr. Robert Hedaya, founder of the Center for Whole Psychiatry & Brain Recovery, explains that restoring physiologic function in the wake of trauma requires healing the gut, supporting the adrenals and liver, and balancing hormones. Modalities like EMDR (eye movement desensitization and reprocessing), EFT (emotional freedom technique), Rolfing, breathwork, and yoga can help change neurological pathways in the brain. Psychedelic-assisted psychotherapy is showing tremendous promise in helping people resolve traumatic experiences.

**Trauma informs care**

Alberta is a twenty-nine-year-old woman whom I met for the first time when she was twenty-four years old. It was years before she shared the multiple traumas she'd experienced in her life. The details trickled out over time.

We first met when she had just finished college. She had been diagnosed with bipolar I and started on lithium and risperidone. She thought the medications triggered hypothyroidism and acne, for which she was started on birth control pills. She felt moody and tired. She described herself as "stress eating" and had gained twenty-five pounds over two years.

Alberta grew up in a home with an alcoholic father. As a child, she felt a lot of pressure to be "incredible." She was accepted into college with a sports scholarship, and, once there, got involved in drugs. After finishing college, she tried to rebalance her life. A two-week episode of not sleeping and constant crying prompted her mom to take her to the hospital. That was when she was diagnosed with bipolar disorder and started on medication.

With time, I recognized Alberta's early and developmental trauma from growing up with an alcoholic parent. Psychiatric hospitalizations and her relationship with her psychiatrist were sources of medical trauma for her. She said on more than one occasion, "I feel like I have no voice in this."

Compounding childhood and medical trauma was Alberta's experience of accumulated stress: she was a primary school teacher throughout the COVID-19 pandemic; she received negative feedback at work; she struggled with her confidence; she felt swamped by medical appointments over the summers.

Aromatherapy and writing provided her the most relief during her tenure with me. She had multiple therapists, none of whom she worked with for very long. She dabbled in EMDR. She tried many psychiatric medications.

The vagus nerve connects the brain, the gut, and the heart. Given the connection of these three organs, it is no surprise that Alberta struggled with gastrointestinal issues, including diarrhea, gas, and reflux. She tried supplements and the Anti-Candida Food Plan, and she did experience some relief from parasite treatment.

Mental, emotional, and spiritual factors profoundly influenced Alberta's health. Was she lucid enough to assess the accuracy of her diagnosis? Sometimes she could follow through with complex treatment plans, and sometimes she could not. Sometimes she experienced a loss of agency in her encounters with the health-care system. She struggled with purpose and whether teaching was the right vocation for her. She felt anger, fear, fatigue, and grief for too many reasons to name here.

Alberta's story is a story unfolding. Her road to health is likely to be long, given her trauma history. She perseveres. I continue to encourage her to do body-based healing and to seek a connection with something bigger than herself.

## Spiritual Health

Patients and I often spend the bulk of our time during office visits discussing matters of the spirit, as these are so often at the core of women's health issues. Spiritual health refers to our sense of meaning and purpose, as well as our relationship with something greater than ourselves. People with a solid relationship with something greater than themselves, whether it be God or the Earth, experience greater levels of health and resilience. My patients have taught me this over and over again. I cared for a woman whose full-term infant died in utero. She went on to labor and birth that baby. Her religious faith was a well of strength for her—it enabled her to carry on and care for her two other young children and supported her through the pregnancy, labor, and birth of a healthy baby. Another woman grew up neglected in a house with a mentally ill mother. I asked her, "Who took care of you?" She said, "Mother Earth." And another woman I cared for through breast cancer quelled her pain and fear through long, silent walks in the woods.

The extent to which women share their adversity, the source of their strength, and their resilience with me makes me feel remarkably privileged. With some frequency, the driving factor that sends a woman's health off the rails is her loss of sense of meaning and purpose. The busyness of life creates a lot of noise, not to mention demands, that can lead us astray. Reconnecting with our meaning and purpose is central to healing, and this is almost always part of our conversation in the clinic.

I once heard the reason people are so drawn to sports is that it provides a way for them to feel connected to something bigger than themselves. I enjoy watching my nephew's Little

League games and the occasional football game on a Sunday afternoon, but I can't say I've ever felt that sports connect me to anything much. I find that connection through the natural world. Give me the wide, open ocean; the beauty of pines against pink granite and a blue sky; or really big mountains. In those places I feel myself as being part of a bigger picture. I don't know if it matters where we find the connection, only that we find it somewhere.

When my daughter, Isabelle, passed, I experienced a spiritual crisis. Prior to her passing, I'd ascribed to the "everything happens for a reason" school of thinking. This philosophy helped me make sense of all kinds of adversity I experienced and witnessed. Adversity does not discriminate based on income, race, class, gender, geography, or any other variable I know of. A lot of famous people have lost children—William Shakespeare, Joe Biden, John Travolta, Mary Tyler Moore, and Vanessa Redgrave, to name a few. It turns out my experience is not all that unique, other than that it is unique to me.

After Isabelle passed, I could not for the life of me figure out what possible reason there could have been for her dying. I've since been able to contrive some possibilities, but I am no longer certain everything happens for a reason. Maybe there is a greater plan—for her, for me—I am not aware of, but that is a tough pill to swallow when your daughter dies.

I did have something to help me keep going, though. I knew from a young age I wanted to work with women. I didn't know the details, per se. Yoga teacher? Naturopath? Physician? I am deeply, deeply grateful for my work. With varying degrees of clarity throughout my life, I have felt my purpose. As my mother-in-law says, everyone needs a reason to get out of bed in the morning. And when I didn't feel like getting out of bed after Isabelle passed, I had my purpose—caring for women—to rise for. It pulled me out of myself, gave me something else to think about, provided me with interaction, and helped me feel like I could, in small bits, despite the pain of life, help someone else feel just a tiny bit better.

Considering and addressing mental, emotional, and spiritual factors is critical to our physical health. Their impact is central to, not separate from, the complex web of our bodies.

# PART TWO

# the nodes of the matrix

# 5

# Converting Fuel to Life

· · · · · · · · · · · · · · · · ·

**ENERGY NODE:** *REGULATION AND MITOCHONDRIAL FUNCTION*

THE CELLS OF *your body convert fats, carbohydrates, and proteins into energy. The process is complex and nutrient dense, meaning it requires a lot of vitamins and minerals, such as B vitamins, zinc, and magnesium. If you don't have enough of these nutrients, you cannot make energy. Low cellular energy production can manifest as fatigue, memory loss, muscle aches, and headaches.*

FATIGUE IS such a common concern for women. It can be complicated getting to *the* root cause because fatigue typically has more than one. Until I started practicing functional medicine, I never considered where energy comes from or the process of energy production in the body.

Mitochondria are the tiny powerhouses, aka organelles, found in most cells where cellular energy production occurs. The biochemical process by which food gets converted into cellular energy is called the Krebs cycle. This arcane process is covered in anatomy and physiology classes, the likes of which I took as a prerequisite for nursing school. I would venture that it is mostly biochemists who remember all the steps and intermediaries involved in the Krebs cycle. Which is to say, it is complex.

What's important for you to know is that the process of energy production within the mitochondria requires *a lot* of nutrients, such as magnesium, zinc, and B vitamins. Without adequate levels of these nutrients, making cellular energy is impossible. Without cellular energy, not only might you feel tired, you might also experience issues such as:

- dementia
- Parkinson's disease
- Alzheimer's disease
- muscle weakness
- heart rate irregularities
- autism
- headaches
- mood disorders

Ensuring there are adequate nutrients to drive energy production is primary in addressing the above health issues.

Working with people with mitochondrial dysfunction takes me to my edge of comfort in clinical practice. Am I really qualified to take care of someone with dementia? Dementia is, or has been made to seem, so medically complex. I'm forthright with patients and their caregivers about the limitations of my knowledge and experience, *and* I am willing to systematically work through the nodes of the matrix to see if I can help. Typically, there is some, even if marginal, improvement.

## Your Cell's Ability to Create Energy

Let's dive a little deeper into the mechanisms of energy production within a cell. Mitochondria are the powerhouses within each cell where most of the chemical energy needed to fuel the cell is made. Cellular energy is called adenosine triphosphate, or ATP.

To optimize energy production, mitochondria require oxygen, macronutrients (protein, fats, carbohydrates), hormones (substances produced to stimulate a specific organ or tissue), peptides (two or more amino acids linked in a chain), neurotransmitters (a chemical messenger from a nerve cell), and growth factors (proteins that promote cell growth). More specifically, mitochondria need oxygen, carbohydrates, proteins, fats, eleven minerals, thirteen vitamins, eight amino acids, and two fatty acids to make ATP. Any deficiency in any one of these requirements can compromise ATP production. When mitochondria fail to produce adequate energy, the result is suboptimal function in the cells within a biologic system.

The work of making energy has a price—the generation of free radicals. Free radicals are unstable molecules that can accumulate in cells and damage other molecules. This increases the risk of disease because when free radicals are not eliminated from the body they cause oxidative stress. Oxidative stress leads to a decline in the body's ability to defend and repair genes, cells, and organs. The products of oxidative damage are called advanced glycation end products, or AGEs. AGEs are ultimately the culprits for what we call "getting old."

Our mother's genes (which solely determine our mitochondrial genetics), our gastrointestinal health, and our nutrient deficiencies influence the efficiency of energy production within our cells. These are antecedents. Triggers affecting energy production include toxins, psychological stress, injury or accident, infection, and inflammation. Mediators affecting energy production include chronic infection, chronic stress, sleep disturbances, and oxidative stress.

Inflammation is the body's defense against injury. The root of the word "inflammation" comes from the Latin word "inflammatio," which means fire. Exposure to bacterial or viral infections, injuries, toxins, and stress trigger the body to release chemicals in an attempt to heal. These chemicals cause a cascade of reactions. When there is acute inflammation, there may be redness, swelling, heat, pain, or loss of function. When there is chronic inflammation, there may be asthma, allergies, or autoimmune disease. Think of inflammation as a fire in your body. You want to stop it before it goes wild.

### The Brain Gets First Dibs

The brain is the first to experience the effects of poor mitochondrial health because this all-important organ gets first dibs on energy in the body. Each brain cell has approximately two million mitochondria. After the brain, energy goes, in order, to the muscles, liver, heart, kidneys, and fat tissue. Each liver cell has over two thousand mitochondria. The liver needs so much energy because detoxification, which largely happens in the liver, requires a lot of energy.

The earliest sign of brain degeneration is brain-based fatigue. Brain-based fatigue occurs with activities that involve activation of the brain such as reading, driving, and other tasks that require thinking. Depression can be the result of early mitochondrial dysfunction. Mild cognitive impairment and Parkinson's and Alzheimer's diseases are examples of severe mitochondrial dysfunction. Imbalances in mitochondria have also been associated with migraines, multiple sclerosis, and epilepsy.

Inflammation crosses the blood-brain barrier, the network of tightly knit cells that keep harmful substances from reaching the brain. Chemical messengers called cytokines activate glial cells in the brain, which causes inflammation. This causes mitochondrial loss, the loss of brain cells (neurons), and a decline in brain function.

Exercise and restricting caloric intake stimulate the production of neurons and good communication between them. This decreases cognitive impairment and slows disease progression. But over-exercising, or metabolic overtraining syndrome, can severely compromise mitochondrial function. Metabolic overtraining syndrome results in decreased antioxidants and increased oxidative stress. Signs and symptoms of overtraining include difficulty finishing an activity or recovering from it, worsening performance, increased injures, decreased motivation and competitive drive, a weakened immune system, decreased sex drive, missed periods, weight increase or loss, and decreased muscle strength. High stress, inflammation, intestinal permeability, hormone imbalance, and obesity predispose someone to metabolic overtraining.

Mitochondria have no defense systems, which leaves them (and you) vulnerable to any substances you ingest or are exposed to. Each of us is responsible for protecting our mitochondria from oxidative stress and the damaging effects of toxins, and for providing them with a nutrient-rich environment.

## Depleted Energy
. . . . . . . . . . . . . . . . . . .

Sixty-eight years old when we first met, Darlene is a petite woman with a big smile and a full heart. She came to her first visit with her husband, who was clearly devoted to her and possibly a bit controlling. Seven years before our meeting, she had been diagnosed with mild cognitive impairment (MCI). Darlene knew her name and where she was. She was uncertain of the day of the week and the date. She sat in a chair for over an hour during that first visit. She tried to answer the questions I asked her and often responded, "I don't know." She remembered some details about her life, but she was unable to articulate what she liked to do for fun.

Differentiating Darlene's earnest dependence on her husband from her husband's tendency to talk over her, correct her, or finish her sentences wasn't easy. Did Darlene really not know what she liked to do for fun, or was it that she couldn't find the language to express it? Her husband knew. He answered for her. Darlene was demure and deferential with me, so gracious for the smallest kindness shown her. Her husband was an avid researcher and was willing to do anything that might help his wife—read, advocate, drive, dance, or cook. We worked together for well over a year. Darlene improved some and taught me a lot. We were partners on her journey to improve her memory.

Darlene did the laundry, the housekeeping, and most of the cooking but was "disorganized." She had difficulty making decisions and following conversations. She had stopped driving a year before I met her. Her goal, as stated by her husband, was for her to be able to drive again.

Unsurprisingly, because everything is connected to everything, MCI was not Darlene's only medical diagnosis. The brain does not exist isolated from the rest of the body. When the brain isn't functioning optimally, other parts of the body are likely

# Energy exists on **a continuum.**

---

to not be functioning optimally either. Darlene had recent cardiac surgery. She had high cholesterol, fibrocystic breasts, and osteopenia. These diagnoses may seem unrelated to MCI, but there is underlying physiology that connects them.

Darlene's family history—family history often being indicative of genetic potential—significantly increased the likelihood of her developing health issues. Her mom died from pancreatic cancer and her dad died in his fifties from a heart attack. He was a heavy drinker. Her sister was diagnosed with fibromyalgia and asbestosis. Her brother had a stroke at forty-five years old and an aortic separation. Based on her family history, Darlene had the genetic potential for cancer and heart disease.

Darlene's husband told me that she enjoyed reading cooking magazines and cookbooks, playing in the kitchen, going to church, and listening to music. She did not drink alcohol or use tobacco, but she did use marijuana daily. She said she slept well. She did not routinely exercise but said she was "on her feet" all day in the kitchen.

I nearly always ask people what they've eaten in the past twenty-four hours, referred to as a "24-hour diet recall." Since food is our first medicine, I am always curious about what a woman eats. Darlene had eaten half an avocado, a piece of provolone, coffee with agave, and green tea. She had butternut squash, rice pilaf, and chicken for dinner the evening prior. She usually ate a sandwich for lunch. She craved salty food and sweets, like dark chocolate. She avoided processed foods, soy lecithin, and fructose. Most of her food was organic. She ate fish once a week and lots of nuts.

## Getting to the Root Cause

I carefully developed Darlene's plan of care. Not only did her decline in memory challenge me, but her recent cardiac surgery added a layer of medical complexity. When we first met, she had yet to start cardiac rehabilitation.

A leaky gut—when the lining of the intestines, which is typically impermeable, becomes permeable such that toxins can move from the intestines into the bloodstream—correlates with a leaky brain. A leaky brain leads to compromised neurological function. I recommended Darlene do food sensitivity testing, as food sensitivities are a common cause of leaky gut. I wanted to identify which foods were inflammatory for her so she could eliminate them from her diet, thereby decreasing inflammation.

Alzheimer's disease is sometimes referred to as type 3 diabetes. Type 3 diabetes occurs when neurons in the brain become unable to respond to insulin. Insulin resistance in the brain is a contributing factor to all neurodegenerative diseases. When there is insulin resistance in the body, it does not typically affect just one organ. It affects all organs and systems because everything is connected to everything. Because of Darlene's diagnosis of MCI and her cardiac history, I was certainly curious to learn if she was eating a large amount of carbohydrates. If she was, it would make sense that the carbohydrates were triggering insulin resistance and insulin resistance was contributing to her cognitive and cardiac dysfunction.

Because of the relationship between elevated cholesterol levels and heart disease, I was curious about Darlene's cholesterol levels. The correlation between insulin resistance and heart disease is actually stronger than cholesterol correlation, but nonetheless, it seemed worthy of evaluation. I was also curious to learn if Darlene tested positive for a genetic marker that is correlated with an increased risk of high cholesterol. I was interested in an in-depth cardiovascular disease assessment that would show us the breakdown of her low-density lipoproteins (LDL), the breakdown of her high-density lipoproteins (HDL), and markers of inflammation, as well as genetic risk markers for high cholesterol, heart disease, and Alzheimer's disease.

I also recommended a Comprehensive Nutritional Evaluation. This measures antioxidants, B vitamins, minerals, amino acids, and fatty acids—the nutrient cofactors necessary to make ATP. This test also looks at markers related to the health of the microbiome and heavy metal toxicity. The results provide specific nutrient recommendations. A custom vitamin and amino acid blend can be formulated. This is the most personalized a supplement regimen can get.

## A Note about Test Results

Test results can be the linchpin in revealing root causes of physiologic imbalances. More often than not, test results serve as a compass, pointing the way. Sometimes, test results are not helpful at all. Too many women come to the clinic saying, "I had my [fill-in-the-blank] tested, and my doctor said my results are normal, but I don't *feel* normal."

There are lots of nuances to consider regarding testing and interpreting test results. Was the testing comprehensive? This is typically *not* the case with thyroid testing. A thyroid stimulation hormone (TSH) level is *not* enough information to get a complete picture about thyroid function. Hormone testing can be tricky to time and interpret depending on whether a woman is menstruating, if she is menstruating regularly, or if she is taking hormones for contraception or post-menopause therapy. There is also the question of what the "best" body fluid is to use to test hormones. Is it blood? saliva? urine? What about the reference range of "normal" used for any particular test? What is normal on paper may not *feel* normal.

Conventional laboratory testing can reveal a lot and is typically accessible through a conventional practitioner. When what can be gleaned from conventional laboratory testing is not enough, there is a world of functional testing available through functional medicine practitioners, naturopaths, and many acupuncturists. I review testing options below and within each of the nodes, conventional and functional, so you can be aware of what exists and get the information you seek.

## ENERGY NODE: CONVENTIONAL LABS

Conventional labs can be ordered by a general practitioner, are conducted at laboratories as part of the conventional medical system, and are typically covered by insurance (depending on your policy, of course).

**Complete blood count (CBC).** A blood test used to evaluate overall health and detect a wide range of disorders including anemia, infection, and leukemia.

**Comprehensive metabolic panel (CMP).** A blood test that measures glucose levels, electrolyte and fluid balance, and kidney and liver function.

**Complete thyroid panel.** Blood tests including thyroid stimulating hormone (TSH), free T3 (FT3), free T4 (FT4), reverse T3 (RT3), thyroid peroxidase antibody (TPOAb), and thyroglobulin antibody (TgAb). Many general practitioners order only a TSH or a TSH and a T4 if the TSH is abnormal. A TSH alone is insufficient information on which to evaluate

Think of inflammation as a fire in your body. **You want to stop it before it goes wild.**

thyroid function. TSH is made in the pituitary gland in the brain. When thyroid levels in the body are low, the pituitary gland makes more TSH. When thyroid levels are high, the pituitary gland makes less TSH. The TSH level can indicate that the thyroid isn't working correctly, but it tells nothing about the availability of active thyroid hormone in the body.

**Ferritin.** A blood test that measures ferritin, the major iron storage protein in the body. Elevated levels may be indicative of inflammation.

**High-sensitivity C-reactive protein (hs-CRP).** A blood test for markers of systemic inflammation. Hs-CRP is a surrogate marker for interleukins, proteins made by white blood cells that regulate immune responses. Hs-CRP screens for infections and inflammatory diseases. It does not diagnose a specific disease.

**Sedimentation rate (sed rate or ESR).** A blood test that reveals inflammatory activity in the body.

### Nutrient markers

These tests measure nutrients most pertinent to the Energy Node.

**Folate.** A blood test measuring all derivatives of folic acid, a marker associated with large red blood cells and anemia. Folate deficiencies are correlated with neurodegenerative disease.

**Vitamin B12.** A blood test that measures levels of B12, a nutrient essential for optimal functioning of the nervous system. B12 helps maintain normal homocysteine levels. Homocysteine is an amino acid that can be tested and is a risk marker for heart disease and inflammation. Homocysteine contributes to glutathione production, and glutathione helps protect cells from damage. B12 also contributes to methylation, one of the ways we eliminate toxins from the body. Testing methlymalonic acid (MMA) is a more accurate way of testing B12 levels (see below).

**Vitamin D3.** A blood test measuring vitamin D3 levels in the body. Two forms of vitamin D are important for nutrition: D2 and D3. Vitamin D2 mainly comes from fortified foods like breakfast cereals, milk, and other dairy items. Vitamin D3 is made by your body when you are exposed to sunlight. It is also found in some foods, including eggs and fatty fish, such as salmon, tuna, and mackerel.

## Metabolites

These labs test for broken-down substances that are specific to the Energy Node.

**Homocysteine.** A blood test that measures this amino acid in the blood. Vitamins B6, B12, and folate are necessary to metabolize homocysteine, such that increased levels of the amino acid may be a sign of deficiency in those vitamins. Homocysteine is also used as a systemic inflammation marker.

**Methylmalonic acid (MMA).** A sensitive and early indicator of B12 deficiency, preferable to a serum B12. MMA is an intermediary in ATP production. I typically test this and a serum B12.

## Infections

Infections profoundly affect energy production on the cellular level. Consider testing for these infections, but know that the presence of these infections does not always correlate with their influence on your health.

**Epstein-Barr virus (EBV).** A blood test for EBV antibodies. Clinical implications of the test results are controversial and vary widely.

**Lyme.** A blood test for Lyme disease. If the results are positive, you have information. Negative results may be because of the lack of sensitivity of the test. Negative Lyme test results may warrant more sensitive testing through a functional laboratory. Lyme is well documented as significantly affecting the nervous system.

### Imaging evaluation methods

These methods produce images of the brain. They help assess head injuries, severe headaches, dizziness, and other symptoms of bleeding, clots, and tumors.

**Computerized axial tomography (CAT scan).** Special imaging that produces cross-sectional images of the brain using X-rays and a computer. This allows images of the inside of the brain to be made.

**Magnetic resonance imaging (MRI).** An imaging technique that uses a magnetic field and radio waves to produce cross-sectional images that allow a view inside the body. Often used to evaluate soft tissues such as the brain, liver, and abdominal organs, as well as to visualize more subtle abnormalities not apparent on regular X-rays.

### ENERGY NODE: FUNCTIONAL LABS

These labs are generally available through functional medicine practitioners, naturopaths, and sometimes acupuncturists. They may or may not be covered partially or fully by conventional insurance policies. Typically people can use their health savings account (HSA), if they have one, to cover the cost.

**Comprehensive Nutritional Evaluation.** A blood and urine test used to evaluate the functional need for antioxidants,

B vitamins, minerals, essential fatty acids, amino acids, digestive support, and other select nutrients. The test also screens for heavy metal toxicity and measures micronutrients essential for optimal ATP production.

**Hydrogen breath test.** A breath test to measure hydrogen and methane, which can be detected through the breath after consuming a specific drink. Elevated levels are indicative of small intestinal bacterial overgrowth (SIBO). This test is available through conventional and functional laboratories. Insurance may cover the cost of the test when processed through a conventional laboratory. The advantage of testing through a functional lab is that the test can be completed at home.

**Stool testing.** A one-day stool collection, done at home, measuring gastrointestinal microbiota DNA. The test detects parasites, bacteria, fungi, and more. It measures indicators of digestion, absorption, inflammation, and immune function.

## Exercise Is a Must

Exercise was a must for Darlene not only for cardiac rehabilitation but also because of the potential benefit to her brain. I requested she consult with her cardiologist for exercise guidelines given her recent surgery.

Exercise increases neuroplasticity, the ability of neurons to reorganize and connect. Neurons that die can be resurrected, in a manner, through neurons that are alive. This restores neurologic function. Exercise also increases nitric oxide. Nitric oxide fuels neurons. And exercise activates the gene that turns on brain-derived neurotrophic factor (BDNF), a protein that protects existing neurons and plays a role in creating new ones. Calorie restriction, curcumin, omega-3 fatty acids, intermittent fasting, intellectual stimulation, and meditation also activate the genes that turn on BDNF.

Two months after her initial visit with me, Darlene had been going to cardiac rehabilitation three times a week for three weeks. She completed all the lab tests I recommended, and we reviewed the results.

I recommended that for three months she eliminate the foods that tested as inflammatory for her on the food sensitivity test. I also recommended she layer an Anti-Candida Food Plan on top of her food eliminations because she tested positive for candida. Candida is one strain of yeast, and yeast overgrowth in the intestines is a common cause of gut imbalance. Yeast is part of our normal body flora, but under certain circumstances it can proliferate and become problematic. It is a common culprit of rectal itching, eczema, constipation, and even depression. We'll take a deeper dive into yeast in chapter 7 when we discuss the Assimilation Node.

Darlene's husband planned to purchase supplements to address the nutrient deficiencies identified on her Comprehensive Nutritional Evaluation. She also started taking probiotics, digestive enzymes, high dose fish oil, methyl folate, CoQ10, and amino acids.

Her cardiologist had prescribed a statin medication, but her cardiovascular disease risk assessment panel showed she had the genetic predisposition to develop muscle weakness while taking statin medications. Darlene's husband planned to work with the cardiologist to stop the statin.

## ENERGY NODE: LIFESTYLE MODIFICATIONS

Lifestyle modifications are actions you can take to affect your health. Adding more to your already long lists of things to do can be overwhelming, so choose one or two changes that you're most inclined toward and start slowly. In general, doing it all—of whatever it is—is tough to maintain. Better to take a baby step, fully integrate it into your life, and then build on that success.

**Exercise.** Exercise improves the function of nearly every node, so you'll see it recommended again and again and again. I recommend thirty minutes of aerobic exercise five days a week, plus two strength-training sessions per week. The greater the intensity of exercise, the more it stimulates neuroplasticity, the ability of the brain to form and make connections between brain cells. Specific to the Energy Node, exercise increases BDNF, the protein that supports neuronal health. Exercise increases oxygenation and improves insulin sensitivity.

**Do new things.** Doing things you've never done before, or do infrequently, increases the development of new neuropathways in the brain.

**Reduce stress.** Like exercise, reducing stress is another recurring recommendation. Diminishing stress reduces cortisol levels, thereby decreasing insulin and insulin resistance, and ultimately preventing type 3 diabetes. Stress reduction also prevents B vitamin depletion.

**Fast intermittently.** Fasting induces ketosis, the production of ketones, when fat, rather than carbohydrates or protein, is used for energy. Ketones are superfood for the brain. Fasting at least twelve hours between dinner and breakfast (or brunch) promotes ketosis. Fasting promotes the destruction of unwanted accumulated molecules. Thin women may not have enough fatty tissue to produce ketones. Adding medium-chain triglyceride (MCT) oil to the diet can aid in ketone production. Fasting for at least three hours prior to going to

**A leaky gut correlates with a leaky brain.** A leaky brain leads to compromised neurological function.

---

bed prevents insulin from inhibiting melatonin and growth hormone, thereby improving sleep and immune function.

**Ensure good sleep.** Sleep induces melatonin, which reduces a protein called amyloid beta. Elevated levels of amyloid beta are associated with Alzheimer's disease. Sleep is critical to memory consolidation, and it removes toxins from the brain.

**Try passive therapies.** Therapies like chiropractic care, aromatherapy, music therapy, craniosacral therapy, massage, and acupuncture improve neurologic function.

### Rebalancing Biochemistry Takes Time

Darlene continued cardiac rehabilitation. When she was done with three months of food eliminations and the Anti-Candida Food Plan, I recommended the Mitochondrial Food Plan developed by IFM. The Mitochondrial Food Plan is designed to support mitochondrial function by providing protective antioxidants, anti-inflammatory nutrients, high-quality dietary fats, low-glycemic impact vegetables, reduced carbohydrates with ketogenic options, intermittent fasting and calorie restriction, and therapeutic foods. It is low grain and gluten-free. This type of plan has been shown to slow the neurodegenerative process. This is using food as medicine.

Darlene's cardiologist changed her statin medication. She modified her supplements. She felt the same, and her husband wasn't noticing a significant difference, but he did note that Darlene seemed more "capable" in the kitchen. I considered this progress. Rebalancing biochemistry takes time.

I requested that Darlene complete a Medical Symptom Questionnaire monthly so we could track her improvement. At her next follow-up, two months later, she stated she was feeling "pretty good." She'd completed cardiac rehabilitation and had cataract surgery. She had a normal bone density test. Through her efforts, she'd reversed her diagnosis of osteopenia.

Bones are essentially a nutrient reservoir. When nutrients from food are not absorbed, the body will send calcium to the bones to transport nutrients out of the bones and into the bloodstream. The body gets what it needs at the bones' expense. For more on this, read *Better Bones, Better Body* by Dr. Susan Brown, or find her online. She is a nutritional anthropologist with a bone health clinic in Syracuse, New York.

Darlene occasionally ate wheat but was avoiding eggs, dairy, and soy completely. She was sleeping well. She was going to a water aerobics class, walking, and stretching. Her husband shared three different occasions when Darlene remembered something. He exuded hope as he shared glimpses of her memory improving.

## ENERGY NODE: NUTRITION INTERVENTIONS

A variety of different strategies to use food as medicine to support the Energy Node exist. Integrate as much or as little as feels right and sustainable for you.

**Try the Mitochondrial Food Plan.** This food plan was developed by IFM. In it, 20 percent of calories come from carbohydrates, 20 percent of calories come from protein, and 60 percent of calories come from fat. The primary source for fuel on the mitochondrial food plan is fat, not glucose. A low carbohydrate–high fat diet leads to b-hydroxylation. B-hydroxybutyrate is superfood for the brain.

**Eat the rainbow.** Eating foods of varying color every day supports all the nodes. Foods rich in color have high levels of antioxidants. The more colorful the foods you consume, the more antioxidants you get. Foods with different colors are phytonutrient rich in different ways. Phytonutrient diversity is key to optimal health. Eating the same foods every day limits nutrient availability. Ask yourself, have I eaten red foods today? orange? yellow? green? For blue foods, think blueberries, blue potatoes, and elderberries; for purple, think purple kale, eggplant, and purple cabbage.

**Incorporate foods that support mitochondrial function.** Consume healthy fats like avocado, salmon, olive oil, and coconut oil (because fat is fuel for the brain); antioxidant-rich foods like spinach, green tea, and blueberries; broccoli and other brassica vegetables (because brassicas help reduce toxins in the body and brain); almonds (because these nuts are rich in omega-3 fatty acids, which are anti-inflammatory and good for the brain); pomegranates; seaweed; and grass-fed beef.

## Supplements

Supplements can support us while we refine our lifestyle and nutrition or compensate for genetic predispositions. Supplements are intended to be *supplemental*. They are not intended to take the place of good nutrition and healthy living. The following nutrients are available as supplements. They provide multiple benefits and have a variety of applications, but they have been included here for their role in optimizing mitochondrial function and energy production.

**B complex.** B vitamins are necessary to fuel the Krebs cycle, the process through which energy is produced, and help preserve memory.

**Choline.** Found in many foods, such as liver, egg yolks, and red meat, and can be taken as a supplement. Choline helps the brain and nervous system regulate memory, mood, and muscle control. Choline also helps form cell membranes.

**CoQ10.** A potent antioxidant that protects and supports mitochondria. CoQ10 plays a central role in the electron transport chain of ATP production.

**Free form amino acids.** Amino acids are required for cellular energy production. It is impossible to make ATP without amino acids. Additionally, amino acids relieve muscle fatigue and assist in recovery from exercise.

**Zinc.** A mineral with antioxidant properties. Deficiency increases reactive oxygen species, which can harm mitochondrial function. Zinc may increase BDNF.

## Root-Cause Resolution Requires a Team

Darlene, her husband, and I worked together for more than a year. She improved some but not enough to satisfy any of us. I referred her to a local chiropractor who specializes in neurodegeneration. I hoped the chiropractor would have different, and more robust, tools to offer Darlene.

I routinely encourage women to seek help from other practitioners. Assembling a health-care team is in your best interest. You need a practitioner who functions within the conventional health-care system who can manage acute medical issues. You may also want a complement of practitioners with a broad range of expertise to address your health from different angles. This does create the risk of "too many cooks in the kitchen." Too many practitioners with too many varying opinions can result in massive, debilitating confusion for patients. But the potential benefit from diverse practitioners with a variety of perspectives and approaches can prove invaluable.

Sure enough, Darlene's chiropractor prescribed walking exercises and exercises to stimulate her vagus nerve. He recommended a few select supplements specific to brain function, and Darlene improved even more. She was reading again and needed less help getting dressed. Darlene continues to resolve the root cause of her MCI.

Root-cause resolution requires full engagement of the practitioner and the patient. It requires a willingness to intervene, assess, reassess, and change course when necessary. This is the art of medicine. There is no one way. There is no right way. The way is determined by an individual's response to an intervention. This requires attentiveness, listening, and an ongoing relationship—not just the doling out of medications and well-wishes for the year. Root-cause resolution requires a team. In this case, physicians who ruled out, or in, pathology; nurse practitioners who took time to teach about leaky gut, leaky brain, and nutrition; and a chiropractor who provided neuro-logic exercises.

Darlene's case illuminates the commitment, patience, and persistence necessary to improve, if not correct, biochemi-cal imbalances. This work is not for the faint at heart. It's not pill-popping and voilà, someone is cured. There is no one pro-tocol. There is no one supplement. There is no one practitioner. Restoration of biochemical imbalance requires a tremendous commitment. Darlene was in part dependent on, and benefited greatly from, her husband's commitment to her wellness.

Energy exists on a continuum, from particle to wave, to mol-ecule, on to cell, organ, organism, local environment, the solar system... Life is ordered energy, ultimately sourced from the sun or Earth. Therefore, planetary health is essential for our ability to make energy efficiently. We are a link in a chain that ultimately creates a circle. Darlene's story exemplifies how sub-optimal cellular energy production leads to suboptimal organ function, which leads to suboptimal function of the person. Her story also shows how nutritional, lifestyle, and nutrient inter-ventions can improve energy production and function.

# 6

# Hormones, Thyroid, and Mood

· · · · · · · · · · · · · · · ·

COMMUNICATION NODE IMBALANCES *are prevalent in our culture for a multitude of reasons related to food choices, lifestyle, and stress. This node is all about how chemical messengers like hormones and neurotransmitters are created and transmitted throughout the body. It encompasses the function of the hypothalamus, pituitary, thyroid, ovarian, and adrenal glands. Premenstrual syndrome, menopause, autoimmune thyroiditis, depression, and anxiety are symptoms and diagnoses that result from imbalances here. For balance in this node, you need to be able to make, use, and eliminate hormones.*

MAINTAINING HORMONE balance over the course of our lives is one of the greatest challenges women face. Hormones are tiny molecules that have huge impact: they are constantly changing, influenced by our genes, what we think, what we eat, how we move, how many hours of sunlight we get in a day, how we manage our stress, and where we are in the childbearing cycle.

Hormones and I go way back. My pursuit of understanding them precedes my becoming a health-care practitioner. I had a pretty normal start to my period at twelve years old. Not too long after, I was stretching in front of a mirror in my mom's bedroom, getting ready for dance class, and then I was on the floor doubled over in pain.

During the harrowing ride to the hospital in the back seat of my mom's car, I was in a lot of pain, and she was frightened. I had a ruptured ovarian cyst, and I was prescribed birth control pills because of it. No one in the emergency room in 1984 talked to me about stress, nutrition, my menstrual cycle, my sexuality, or any of the other topics that might contribute to ovarian cyst production.

Ultimately, I stopped the birth control pills because I did not want to take hormones, despite having severe menstrual cramps that occasionally kept me bedridden for a few days. In my early twenties, I began to connect the dots between my high carbohydrate, vegetarian diet and the severity of my menstrual cramps. I used herbs, exercise, food, and ibuprofen to manage the pain with good results.

I had a particularly difficult time after the birth of my son. I struggled with my mood in the winter. I did not understand at the time that these experiences are related and are a frequent and observable pattern in women with hormone imbalance.

In my midwifery training, I was taught that women either have hormones or they don't. If a woman had low hormones, all you had to do was replace them and presumably she would feel better—except that often she didn't. If she had too many hormones, all you had to do was block the production of them and she would feel better—except that often she didn't. It turns out, achieving hormone balance is not as simple as "add some" or "take some away."

I didn't understand the complexity of balancing hormones until I started practicing functional medicine. In 2006, I attended the hormone module through IFM and learned about the pathways of hormone production. I had been practicing women's health for seven years by that time. At that course, I learned that cholesterol is the biochemical precursor for making hormones and that having low cholesterol (which can be the case for various reasons, the most common being taking statin medication to treat high cholesterol) is a significant contributor to hormone imbalance. I learned about how our genes influence how we detoxify our hormones and what that means in terms of our risk of cancer. I learned about which foods to eat to support hormone balance, the influence of exercise on hormone balance, and how important it is to regularly move the bowels so estrogen stored in the stool isn't reabsorbed into the bloodstream. Hormones in poop: it's a thing.

## Insulin and Hormone Balance

Understanding the role of insulin is critical to understanding hormone balance (and a lot of other things, too, that you will read about in the different nodes). Insulin is a hormone produced in the pancreas. It helps our bodies control the levels of glucose (sugar) in our blood. When the body cannot make enough insulin to respond to what we eat, or the body's response to insulin is impaired, the result is elevated levels of glucose in the blood. Elevated blood glucose is a key component of:

- type 2 diabetes
- metabolic syndrome
- mid-section weight gain
- polycystic ovarian syndrome (PCOS)
- many other hormone imbalances

"Insulin resistance" or "insulin block" is the term used to describe when cells in muscles, fat, and the liver do not respond well to insulin. The body cannot take up glucose from the blood. In turn, the pancreas makes more insulin in an effort to get glucose into the cells. The insulin levels grow higher and higher, yet the tissues are not getting the glucose they need to function well. Insulin resistance slows metabolism, increases inflammation, causes cravings, and creates fat storage.

Additionally, when insulin levels are high, less sex hormone binding globulin (SHBG) is made. SHBG is a protein produced in the liver that binds to three sex hormones: estrogen, dihydrotestosterone, and testosterone. SHBG controls the amount of these hormones that is delivered to the body's tissues. High insulin leads to low SHBG, which leads to high levels of hormones in the bloodstream.

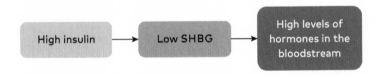

We can do a lot to improve our body's response—or sensitivity—to insulin:

- exercise, particularly strength training
- reduce stress
- improve sleep

- decrease carbohydrate intake
- decrease sugar intake
- eat more fiber
- eat the rainbow
- add cinnamon
- drink green tea
- supplement with chromium, magnesium, berberine, or resveratrol

Remember that when stress levels are high, often cortisol levels are high. When cortisol levels are elevated, insulin levels are elevated.

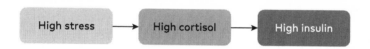

This is how stress contributes to insulin resistance. Managing stress, thereby reducing cortisol levels, helps regulate blood sugar and, subsequently, hormone balance. Let that sink in.

The ovaries, the adrenals, and the thyroid are on the same hormone axis. The hypothalamus and pituitary, parts of the brain, are also part of the axis. This is referred to as the HPTAG axis (hypothalamic, pituitary, thyroid, adrenal, gonadal—the latter of which, in women, are the ovaries). What affects one organ affects the other. When the adrenals are working to manage stress, you may have thyroid or hormone symptoms. When your ovaries are working, either because you are getting your period or losing your period or you just had a baby, imbalances in the adrenals or thyroid may arise. This is referred to as HPTAG axis dysfunction. Intervening on any level alleviates stress in the whole system. For example, managing stress

**It is simply unrealistic** to neglect ourselves and expect to feel well.

———————

profoundly improves hormone imbalances. Everything is connected to everything.

Ovaries are the primary production site of our sex hormones—think estrogen, progesterone, and testosterone. The adrenals, small glands that sit on top of your kidneys and are primarily responsible for the production of cortisol, also make some sex hormones, specifically DHEA, which is a precursor to testosterone. A woman who has had a total hysterectomy will still have some sex hormone production from her adrenal glands.

The thyroid is considered a sentinel gland. It stands and keeps watch over the entire body. The thyroid has a part in controlling all physiologic functions including body temperature, weight, mood, and energy. You have thyroid receptor cells in nearly every organ in your body. Many nutrients, including vitamin D3, selenium, and iodine, contribute to thyroid function and hormone production. The extent to which your cells receive thyroid hormone is influenced by multiple lifestyle factors including stress and exercise.

## Hormone Balance Differs through Every Stage of Life

Women go about hormone balance in a whole variety of ways. Some women want balance regardless of their lifestyle, and others tailor their lifestyle for hormone balance but still need support. Elements of hormone balance remain mysterious. Is hormone balance tied to the season? to the phases of the moon? to the land on which we live?

Some of the reasons a conventional approach to hormone balance may be ineffective are as follows:

* Some hormone medications differ from the hormones we make in our bodies. These medications are metabolized in a way that can increase adverse health effects.

- Conventional medicine often fails to address nutrition as crucial for hormone balance. For example, cholesterol is the precursor to hormone production. A woman who has low cholesterol, maybe because she eats a low-fat diet or because she is taking a statin medication for high cholesterol, may experience symptoms of hormonal imbalance.

- Our genes influence how we break down our hormones.

- Women need different levels of hormones to feel well.

- Modulating stress is critical for hormone balance.

- What women need for hormone balance is different during different stages of life.

Some functional medicine practitioners insist women optimize their adrenal gland function, meaning manage their stress, prior to providing hormone support. In theory, I agree. In practice, sometimes women benefit from hormone support so they can do what needs doing to get well, not *instead* of modulating stress but in addition to it.

Hormone imbalance presents in a multitude of ways. Young women may experience:

- no periods
- irregular periods
- constant periods
- premenstrual syndrome
- PCOS
- endometriosis

Too often, young women are put on birth control pills without ever being taught how lifestyle and nutrition affect hormone balance. But this information can empower young women to do what they can to avert the snowball of hormone imbalance that can accumulate throughout a lifetime.

The childbearing years pose their own hormonal challenges:

- fertility issues
- pregnancy
- postpartum depression
- contraception

Common concerns of middle-aged women who present to the clinic include, but are not limited to, imbalances they have carried since their younger years, such as:

- endometriosis

- polycystic ovaries, or fibroids

- perimenopause (the time leading up to menopause, which by definition is a year without a period) with all of its associated symptoms (worsening premenstrual syndrome, anxiety, insomnia, low sex drive, weight gain, heavy bleeding, and fatigue)

- gynecologic cancers (which often appear during this stage of life as the hormone imbalance accumulates)

A patient once said to me, "I hate the word 'menopause.' I refuse to use it. I'm calling it turbulence." *I love this.* Midlife can feel quite turbulent. You may want to fasten your seatbelt.

Well tended, midlife is a transition, not a crisis. But by midlife, your body manifests the net result of self-neglect as you were busy doing other things like raising careers or families. Your body insists you take care of yourself, lest you feel horrible. This is actually quite beautiful, although it can bring you to your knees. You do have some choice and control, however. And while you may not be able to drink wine like you used to, giving it up may be a worthy concession for a decent night of sleep and less belly fat.

Many a seventy-year-old woman comes to the clinic fanning her face as she has a hot flash, asking, "What the heck is this about, Carrie? I haven't had a period in twenty years." My response: Menopause is not a one-way train with a destination where you hop off. It's common for menopausal symptoms to recur, especially during periods of high stress like the death or illness of a loved one. Some older women seek support because they are in new relationships and want to resume sexual activity but feel physically unable. Some women come because they want to do all they can to age well.

There is an observable pattern of hormone imbalance in women. It starts with issues around menstruation in the younger years, premenstrual syndrome, maybe a diagnosis of endometriosis or polycystic ovaries, maybe issues with fertility, seasonal affective disorder, postpartum depression, a turbulent midlife transition, and the possibility of a gynecologic cancer along the way. Very rarely does a woman present with hormone concerns and no previous history of hormone imbalance. Too often, along her way she had symptoms of hormone imbalance that were treated with medication, not resolved—hence the snowball.

Brain fog, weight-loss resistance, and hair loss often manifest as a result of Communication Node imbalance. Other imbalances that fall within the Communication Node include thyroid and neurotransmitter imbalances. Diagnoses that fall within the Communication Node include hypothyroidism, hyperthyroidism, autoimmune thyroid disease (including autoimmune thyroiditis and Graves' disease), depression, and anxiety.

## Hormone Imbalance Manifested

Andrea was a forty-two-year-old mother of three when we first met. She had a strong Christian faith and homeschooled her kids. Her concerns were a typical laundry list of symptoms—premenstrual syndrome, depression, and weight gain. She experienced cyclic anxiety. She'd had a partial hysterectomy, so she still had her ovaries but not her uterus, which meant she still cycled but no longer bled. Surgical menopause or a partial hysterectomy muddies the bounds of menopause. With a partial hysterectomy, many women report feeling their cycle even during menopause. The ovaries do not have an "off" switch, and the adrenals will continue to produce sex hormones for as long as they are able. When symptoms have a monthly, cyclic pattern, that is a clue that hormones may be imbalanced. Andrea felt the stress of homeschooling her children, managing her household, and maintaining community involvement. Like so many midlife women, she struggled to give herself a piece of the time and energy she gave to her family.

Andrea's medical history included irregular periods, with heavy bleeding and painful cramps; adenomyosis, a condition when the tissue that normally lines the uterus grows into the muscular wall of the uterus; years of premenstrual syndrome treated with Zoloft; and a partial hysterectomy. Her symptoms had been managed with medicine over the years, but because the root of her physiologic imbalance hadn't been corrected, she still experienced symptoms of hormone imbalance. She was also diagnosed with autoimmune thyroiditis—which came as no surprise because we are whole and our physiologic systems are connected.

I was curious about Andrea's thyroid function, her hormones, and her insulin and blood sugar levels. I wanted to know if she was eating too many carbohydrates, because of the relationship between insulin resistance and hormone imbalance.

We tested Andrea's thyroid because of her documented thyroid disease. We tested her fasting insulin and glucose levels to see if she was insulin resistant. We tested her hemoglobin A1C (HgA1C) to get a bigger picture of her blood sugar stability over the past three months. We tested her vitamin D3 to see if a deficiency might be part of her depression. We opted against testing her hormones because of the absence of her period. Without a period, it is difficult to determine normal levels of hormones because they change throughout the cycle. Andrea was aware of the cyclic nature of her symptoms and anticipated when they would get better and worse throughout the month.

### COMMUNICATION NODE: CONVENTIONAL LABS

**Complete thyroid panel.** Blood tests including thyroid stimulating hormone (TSH), free T3 (FT3), free T4 (FT4), reverse T3 (RT3), thyroid peroxidase antibody (TPOAb), and thyroglobulin antibody (TgAb). Many general practitioners order only a TSH or a TSH and a T4 if the TSH is abnormal. A TSH alone is insufficient information on which to evaluate thyroid function. TSH is made in the pituitary gland in the brain. When thyroid levels in the body are low, the pituitary gland makes more TSH. When thyroid levels are high, the pituitary gland makes less TSH. The TSH level can indicate that the thyroid isn't working correctly, but it tells nothing about the availability of active thyroid hormone in the body. Thyroid peroxidase antibody and thyroglobulin antibodies are markers for autoimmune thyroiditis also known as Hashimoto's disease.

**Managing stress helps regulate** blood sugar and, subsequently, hormone balance.

———————————

**Fasting and two-hour insulin and glucose.** A blood test measuring insulin and glucose levels first thing in the morning before eating and again after consuming a large amount of carbohydrates. Consuming a large amount of carbohydrates challenges the pancreas to make enough insulin to metabolize the carbohydrates. This blood test is the gold standard used to diagnose insulin resistance and type 2 diabetes.

**HgA1c.** A blood test measuring blood sugar stability over the past three months.

**Homocysteine.** A blood test that measures this amino acid in the blood. Vitamins B6, B12, and folate are necessary to metabolize homocysteine, such that increased levels of the amino acid may be a sign of deficiency in those vitamins.

**Methylenetetrahydrofolate reductase (MTHFR).** A blood test that can detect the two most common mutations of the MTHFR gene, which contain the code to produce the MTHFR enzyme. The enzyme is critical for metabolizing one form of B vitamin, folate, into another.

**Sex hormone binding globulin (SHBG).** A blood test measuring SHBG, a protein made in the liver. SHBG controls how much estrogen and testosterone are delivered to the body's tissues.

**Vitamin D3.** A blood test measuring vitamin D3 levels in the body. Two forms of vitamin D are important for nutrition: D2 and D3. Vitamin D2 mainly comes from fortified foods like breakfast cereals, milk, and other dairy items. Vitamin D3 is made by your body when you are exposed to sunlight. It is also found in some foods, including eggs and fatty fish, such as salmon, tuna, and mackerel. Vitamin D3 functions more like a hormone than a vitamin. It has been shown to significantly decrease symptoms of depression.

## COMMUNICATION NODE: FUNCTIONAL LABS

**2-, 4-, 16alpha-hydroxyestrone.** A urine test that measures the metabolites 2-, 4-, and 16alpha-hydroxyestrone. Estrogen is metabolized first in the gut and then in the liver. In the liver, estrogen gets broken down into 2-, 4-, and 16alpha-hydroxyestrone. These metabolites are markers related to increased risk of estrogen-related diseases or disease protection against estrogen-related diseases. If you know your body is breaking down estrogen in a way that increases your risk of estrogen-dependent diseases, you can influence that process with things like exercise, flaxseed, and eating cruciferous vegetables.

**Comprehensive Nutritional Evaluation.** A blood and urine test used to evaluate the functional need for antioxidants, B vitamins, minerals, essential fatty acids, amino acids, digestive support, and other select nutrients. The test also screens for heavy metal toxicity and measures micronutrients essential for optimal ATP production. Amino acids are necessary for neurotransmitter production, neurotransmitters being hormones that regulate mood.

**Cortisol.** A blood, urine, or saliva test. Salivary and urine cortisol testing can be done at home and measure cortisol levels at four different times over twenty-four hours. Conventional medical practitioners typically measure cortisol in the blood and acknowledge two diseases of the adrenal gland: Cushing's syndrome is a condition that causes the body to make too much cortisol, and Addison's disease is a condition in which the body doesn't make enough cortisol. Functional practitioners acknowledge adrenal dysfunction that exists between the extremes of too much or too little cortisol production.

**Genomic testing.** A sample of cells from the cheek used to identify single nucleotide polymorphisms (SNPs) associated with increased risk of impaired detoxification capacity, related to either environmental toxins or hormone metabolism. Genetic expression is significantly influenced by the environment in which genes live. Particular to the Communication Node, saliva testing for genes specific to hormone metabolism can be evaluated. Nutrition, lifestyle, and supplements can leverage the activity of genes.

**Hormone testing.** Serum, blood spot, urine, and saliva testing to measure hormone levels. Testing hormone levels through serum and urine are the best methods for women who are menstruating. Serum testing is done on days three and twenty-one of the menstrual cycle. This testing is generally covered by insurance and gives a cursory insight into hormone levels. The results are limited because they provide information from only two days in a cycle, which may not accurately reflect fluctuations throughout the cycle. A better choice for testing hormone levels in a menstruating woman is to use a urine test done at home with multiple samples collected over the course of the month. Multiple data points create a clearer picture of hormone levels throughout a woman's cycle.

Because of fluctuating hormone levels, testing serum hormone levels during perimenopause is of limited value. Cycles during perimenopause are often irregular, so determining a reference range of normal for a particular hormone is near impossible. The same is true for women who are not menstruating at all. Without knowing where she is in her cycle, making sense of hormone levels is challenging.

Many women believe they are menopausal based on having had their follicle stimulating hormone (FSH) and estradiol levels measured. A menstruating person is *not* menopausal, regardless of an elevated FSH or low estradiol. From a laboratory perspective, menopause is defined as a serum FSH over 80 and a serum estradiol level of less than 20, but these values can occur in a woman who is *peri*menopausal.

The information from urine testing is comprehensive in that it provides information about estrogen metabolites. See 2-, 4-, 16alpha-hydroxyestrone above.

## How Lifestyle Impacts Hormones

Andrea and I talked a lot about her lifestyle—her nutrition, her exercise, her sleep, her relationships, and her fun, or lack thereof. She wasn't exercising at all because she didn't feel she had enough time. Many women feel they don't have enough time to exercise. We don't have enough time to *not* exercise.

No pill can do for our health what exercise does. It's not a matter of having time for exercise, it's a matter of *making* time. No one is ever going to clear your schedule for you so that you have the time to exercise. You have to put a stake in the ground for exercise and work the day around it. When my kids were little, a large part of why I didn't work five days a week was that I couldn't figure out how to juggle home and work responsibilities and exercise all in the same day.

Starting slow with exercise seems to yield positive results. It's likely to be unrealistic to expect to go from no exercise to exercising five days a week. If you are new to exercise or newly returning, start with short sessions at infrequent intervals. Small steps can produce big rewards and are typically sustainable. You can then build on your success.

I asked Andrea if she felt she could carve out time for two ten-minute walks a week. She and I talked about her getting some help homeschooling her kids so she might have a bit of personal time. She loved to knit but rarely took the time to do so. I encouraged her to take some of her respite time and spend it doing what she loved.

## COMMUNICATION NODE:
## LIFESTYLE MODIFICATIONS

**Be mindful of your carbohydrate intake.** I am not necessarily an advocate of eliminating carbohydrates, which is, frankly, impossible to do, as most food has some carbohydrates in it. Some women do feel best with no grains. I like what Dr. Mark Hyman says: "It's not no carbs, it's slow carbs." I understand this to mean we need not eliminate all carbohydrates, but we are better off consuming complex carbohydrates. Limit simple carbohydrates such as milk, large amounts of fruit, sugar, and foods made with white flour. Enjoy complex carbohydrates such as starchy vegetables, whole grains, and beans. Our ability to metabolize carbohydrates decreases as we age, and we need fewer of them.

Midsection weight gain—the much loathed "muffin-top"—suggests the consumption of too many carbohydrates or elevated levels of stress hormones. Decreasing carbohydrate intake, particularly simple carbohydrates like bread, cereal, pasta, processed foods, and desserts, could be the single largest lifestyle intervention positively affecting every node in the matrix.

**Poop every day.** At least once. Pooping is the primary mechanism for eliminating the by-products, or toxins, of hormone metabolism. You don't want those toxins sitting in your colon, where they can be reabsorbed into the bloodstream. Ideally, poop should be a soft, formed stool with narrow, tapered ends.

**Sweat.** Sweat is another key mechanism by which we eliminate toxins, like hormone metabolites, from our bodies. Aerobic exercise, hot yoga, Epsom salt and baking soda baths, and saunas all promote sweating.

**Exercise.** Exercise that is part of daily living, such as climbing stairs, house cleaning, gardening, or walking for transportation, may not be enough to modulate hormone imbalance. I recommend thirty minutes of aerobic exercise five days a week, plus two strength-training sessions per week. Exercise raises serotonin, promotes sweating and detoxification, improves muscle mass, and promotes intestinal motility. It improves sleep, reduces stress, reduces fat, and improves insulin sensitivity—all supporting Communication Node imbalances.

**Rest.** No supplement on the planet restores adrenal gland function the way rest does.

## Eating Well for Hormone Health

Andrea shared her lifelong history of eating for comfort. She felt this was a significant barrier to her eating well. Like so many of us, it's not that she didn't *know* how to eat well, it's that she felt *unable* to do it. She also did not like vegetables. I encouraged her to work with a counselor on her emotional eating. I also recommended a greens supplement to compensate for her not eating many vegetables.

Andrea and I both knew that without a toolbox full of strategies to help her manage her eating, she would inevitably bump into a situation in life that would compel her to make less-than-ideal food choices. In addition to counseling, I suggested Andrea use the Core Food Plan developed by IFM as a foundation for healthy eating. The Core Food Plan takes elements from the Mediterranean diet and the hunter-gatherer approach.

You have to be able to make, use, and eliminate hormones **to have hormone balance.**

———————————

The major focus of the plan is replacing processed food with vegetables, fruits, nuts, seeds, legumes, whole grains, anti-inflammatory fats, and high-quality protein. IFM has a suite of food plans that provide fantastic structure, including grocery lists, menu plans, and recipes that are accessible through functional medicine practitioners.

## COMMUNICATION NODE:
## NUTRITION INTERVENTIONS

**Eat brassicas.** Common brassicas are broccoli, cauliflower, brussels sprouts, cabbage, turnips, collards, kale, arugula, and bok choy. Brassicas are rich in sulforaphane, indole-3-carbinol, and diindolylmethane (DIM), phytonutrients (plant nutrients) that promote healthy estrogen metabolism. They are also rich in fiber that supports the production of short-chain fatty acids, essential for a healthy microbiome. Fiber also supports regular bowel movements and helps stabilize blood sugar levels.

**Eat seeds.** Seeds are high in fiber and rich in omega-3 fatty acids. Fiber helps detoxify hormones. Some seeds are thought to be high in estrogen and others in progesterone. Some women improve their hormone balance through seed cycling. The follicular phase is the first two weeks of the menstrual cycle, during which time women consume one tablespoon each of flax and pumpkin seeds every day. Flax and pumpkin seeds are rich in phytoestrogens, plant sources of estrogen capable of producing estrogenic effects. The luteal phase is the last two weeks of the menstrual cycle, during which time women consume one tablespoon each of sunflower and sesame seeds a day. Sunflower and sesame seeds are thought to boost progesterone production. Progesterone staves off symptoms of premenstrual syndrome.

**Eat soy.** Soy is a phytoestrogenic food, meaning it is a plant-based source of estrogen. Consuming soy can remedy symptoms of low estrogen such as hot flashes and night sweats. Current research shows that soy does not increase the risk of estrogen-dependent cancers because it binds to non-cancer receptors. Research also shows that normal, dietary consumption of soy is safe for people with thyroid disease. A little bit of non-GMO tofu, tempeh, or edamame may offer hormone support and is a vegetarian source of protein.

**Eat fat.** Fat is the biochemical precursor to cholesterol, which is the biochemical precursor to pregnenolone, which is the biochemical precursor to progesterone and all the other sex hormones. Hormone balance requires healthy fat consumption from salmon, avocadoes, nuts, and oils. Healthy fats do not make us fat, excess carbohydrates do.

**Eat berries.** Berries are nutrient dense, rich in antioxidants, vitamins, minerals, and soluble fiber. They also have a low glycemic index, which means they don't elevate blood sugar and insulin levels like fruits with a high glycemic index (bananas, for example). Goji berries are the most nutrient dense of all the berries followed by black raspberries.

## Supplements

**5-hydroxytryptophan (5-HTP).** The biochemical precursor to serotonin (the antidepressant neurotransmitter), 5-HTP supports mood and sleep and has been shown to decrease food cravings.

**Bioidentical plant-based progesterone cream.** Progesterone can help alleviate postpartum depression, depression, premenstrual syndrome, and perimenopausal symptoms. It can leverage symptoms of estrogen dominance, which is when there are high levels of estrogen relative to low levels of pro-gesterone. Bioidentical plant-based progesterone is available over the counter as a topical cream, and although many conventional practitioners are uncomfortable with the use of bioidentical hormone therapy, it is a low-risk intervention and frequently quite helpful.

**Calcium D-glucarate.** A chemical similar to naturally occurring glucaric acid, which is found in the body as well as in fruits and vegetables. Calcium D-glucarate combines glucaric acid with calcium. It supports the body's defense against toxins and excess steroid hormones. Calcium D-glucarate may lower estrogen levels and can be used when symptoms of excess estrogen are present.

**CoQ10.** A potent antioxidant that declines with age. Low levels of CoQ10 are associated with hormone imbalance.

**DIM.** A compound derived from the digestion of indole-3-carbinol, found in cruciferous vegetables like kale and broccoli. DIM helps rid the body of excess estrogen and may support healthy estrogen metabolism.

**Omega-3 fatty acids.** Essential fats the body can't make but must get from food or supplementation. They are part of the cell membrane and affect the function of the receptors in cell membranes. They modulate contraction, relaxation, inflammation, and gene function. They decrease joint pain and inflammation. Omega-3 fatty acids are one of the building blocks for hormone production, and they reduce inflammation and help stabilize blood sugar, all of which supports hormone and mood stability.

**Selenium.** A group of enzymes called seleniumases, made with selenium, are required for thyroid hormone conversion. Brazil nuts are rich in selenium.

**Vitamin B12.** Supplementation is suggested for women who are vegetarian, taking birth control pills, or have a documented deficiency. B12 deficiencies are implicated in a variety of health issues, including hormone and mood imbalances. B12 declines as we age, largely because of the decline in hydrochloric acid in our stomach. Hydrochloric acid is necessary to cleave B12 from dietary intake of meat.

## Restoring Physiological Balance

Repairing physiologic imbalances within the Communication Node requires:

* normal cortisol levels
* blood sugar stability
* micronutrient and amino acid sufficiency
* functional detoxification pathways
* adequate hormone production and cellular receptivity to hormones

Adding or removing hormones simply does not get the job done.

Andrea's symptoms of premenstrual syndrome, depression, and weight gain were significantly improved by her efforts. But her efforts did not come easily. She worked to make time for exercise and to do some of what she loved beyond caring for her family and her community. She increased her exercise to thirty minutes four times a week. She continued to work with her counselor on emotional eating. She explored vegetables and methods of preparing them in hope that she would someday enjoy them. She learned that vegetables are essential to her health. She took and continues to take supplements, augmenting her efforts to live a more balanced life.

It is simply unrealistic to neglect ourselves and expect to feel well. When we hear ourselves talk out loud about all we are up against, what we are doing about it, and how horrible we feel, the path to wholeness often becomes crystalline. Establishing a team of practitioners in support of our efforts is often the difference between success and failure, health and disease.

If you are eating well, have a sound lifestyle, and still are not feeling well—I see you. I hear your frustration. Sometimes, good nutrition and healthy living are not enough to correct significant physiologic imbalances. This reality can feel maddening. Who wants to work hard with little result for any length of time? Testing can be helpful in this situation. An intrepid, seasoned practitioner can be helpful too—someone who is willing to look in the nooks and crannies for an explanation of what is going on.

Medications for hormone, thyroid, and mood support have their time and place, but not in lieu of tending to the pathways involved in making, using, and getting rid of hormones. Medication is a tool in the toolbox, supporting us while we work out the lifestyle parts of the matrix. Tending to the pathways prevents physiologic imbalance from arising in a different body part in a different way. This is preventative health care at its best.

# 7

# Digesting, Pooping, and All Things Microbiome

· · · · · · · · · · · · · · · ·

**ASSIMILATION NODE:** *DIGESTION,*
*ABSORPTION, MICROBIOTA AND*
*GASTROINTESTINAL TRACT, RESPIRATION*

INTESTINAL HEALTH *is essential for overall health and wellness. The food you eat interacts with your entire body through the lymph tissue lining the intestines. When you eat an inflammatory food, the inflammation is communicated from your gut to the bloodstream, triggering a series of biochemical reactions that then circulate throughout your body. Inflammation you feel in your heel—or shoulder or sinuses or skin or bladder or uterus—may have roots in your gut. Gastrointestinal issues like irritable bowel syndrome, gas, and bloating are more obvious symptoms of imbalances here. Less obvious symptoms include rashes, depression, asthma, and allergies.*

WHEN I FIRST started practicing functional medicine, my mentor said, "If you don't know where to start, start with the gut." I follow this guidance to this day. The reverberations of imbalances of the Assimilation Node are extensive. When I start with the gut, a patient's health inevitably improves in some way. The first book I read when I started training at Women to Women was *Digestive Wellness* by Elizabeth Lipski. Reading that book was like taking off one pair of glasses and putting on a new pair. *Digestive Wellness* forever changed the way I understand health. Conditions like fibromyalgia, irritable bowel syndrome, chronic fatigue syndrome, and even schizophrenia, conditions that conventional medicine historically has had little to offer save medication, were completely reframed in my mind through reading this book. Most of my patients come to me not understanding the centrality of gut health to overall health and wellness. Multiple conditions can be related to it, including:

- insomnia
- anxiety
- rashes
- fibromyalgia
- joint pain
- muscle pain
- skin eruptions (psoriasis, eczema, rosacea)
- irritable bowel syndrome
- bloating
- acid reflux
- diarrhea
- constipation

What we eat matters. A *lot*. What we put in our mouths is the single largest variable within our control to positively or negatively affect our health. One would think this is obvious given the Standard American Diet (SAD—the lethal combination of eating lots of carbohydrates, processed sugar, and saturated fats) and the high incidences of chronic disease and illness, such as obesity, high cholesterol, high blood pressure, and heart disease, related to this manner of eating.

Eating vegetables is the name of the game for optimizing gut health. Vegetables provide vitamins and minerals that we cannot get from other foods. Organisms living in our gut ferment the fiber from vegetables (and some complex carbohydrates) and produce short-chain fatty acids (SCFAs). SCFAs are the primary source of energy for cells in our intestines. Without SCFAs, we cannot have normal bowel movements or an intact immune system.

The majority of our immune system is in our gut. The tissue lining the gut, mucosa-associated lymphatic tissue (MALT), which is found in submucosal membranes throughout the body, including the nose, thyroid, breast, lungs, salivary glands, eyes, and skin, and gut-associated lymphoid tissue (GALT), which is the component of MALT specific to the gut, comprises a large component of our immune system. When gut health is compromised, the immune system is compromised. So, when a woman comes to the clinic with the diagnosis of an autoimmune disease, or four—because once that physiologic process starts, if it isn't stopped, it steamrolls through the body—I am less concerned about *which* specific autoimmune disease she has. It's enough for me to know that her immune system is activated and the home of the immune system is in the gut.

Dairy and gluten, a protein found in wheat, rye, oats, and barley, are the most common dietary agents of inflammation contributing to gut imbalance. Dairy and gluten are similar, and often the body cannot differentiate between the two. Which is why if a woman tells me she's tried eliminating either gluten *or* dairy without effect, I generally recommend she try eliminating *both* foods to see if her symptoms improve. Grains in general, not just wheat, trigger inflammation for a growing number of people. Some women feel best eliminating most, if not all, grains.

Why gluten and dairy? Why so many people? The answer is complicated. The issue with gluten may be related to the way wheat is grown in America. Many women report they cannot tolerate gluten here, but when they travel abroad, they tolerate it without difficulty. The prevalence of gluten and dairy sensitivity may be related to the sheer volume of these foods that are consumed as part of the SAD. Much of our American culture depends on grab-and-go food. Too many women tell me they eat in the car as they commute or shuttle children around. We, as a culture, don't take time to eat, to sit down and nourish ourselves, let alone savor what we are eating. I'll never forget my kids' first experience of candy. They were sitting still. It was otherwise quiet in the room. It was a full sensory experience of pleasure. In that moment, I learned that the environment in which we consume our food influences our emotional experience of it and our body's reaction to it.

Agribusiness and the use of pesticides as well as the quality of the soil food is grown in affect the quality of the food we eat. The quality of food we have access to is influenced significantly by our socioeconomic status: Processed foods are less expensive than whole foods. Preparing food also takes an equipped kitchen, time, and energy—resources not everyone has. Then there is *knowing* what to do with a particular food. If you grew up in a home where meals were mostly takeout, cooking is a skill you may not have acquired. Some people simply don't enjoy cooking.

It's no wonder that gut health and food and nutrition are complicated. So many forces are at work, not to mention the confusion people experience about what is "good" to eat. I recently read two women's health books, both published in

2021, one pro intermittent fasting and the other against it. This goes to show that there is no one best way of eating that is good for everyone.

A patient told me the story of growing up on a farm with cows and a giant vegetable garden. Her family was poor, so they ate what they grew and raised. As a kid, she envied her friends who got to eat TV dinners, which were considered a sign of affluence and "better than" food that came from the earth. I remember those TV dinners—the turkey, the pasty gravy, the sweet cranberry sauce. I loved them. By way of her upbringing, this patient learned to freeze and can vegetables. She loves food that comes from the earth and is bemused by the irony that now, food that comes from the earth is most accessible to those with the economic means to afford it.

I recommend that, once your gut is healed, you eat a modified Mediterranean diet—lots of vegetables, lean protein, complex carbohydrates, nuts, seeds, beans, and healthy fats. You never have to read another diet book again. There are nuances, of course, depending on your health. But if you need a general recommendation, here it is.

Fill half your plate with vegetables. Fill one quarter of your plate with complex carbohydrates, such as sweet potato, brown rice, or starchy vegetables such as winter squash or corn. Fill the last quarter of your plate with lean protein—grass-fed beef, turkey, fish, chicken, pork, tofu, or beans. Put your scale away. Weighing food at every meal is unsustainable behavior. It may be therapeutic for a time, but it is not a lifestyle. Nor is deprivation. And weighing yourself every day is a sure path to discontentment. If you are compelled to weigh yourself, limit it to once a week. Most of us know when our pants feel good and when they feel too snug.

As a general rule, eat food that comes from the earth 80 percent of the time. The other 20 percent of the time, eat whatever you want—except artificial sweeteners. More on that later. I know people for whom eating is about sustenance alone. Kudos to them. I was raised in a house where food was love, and for me, food is love made visible. It is one of the biggest ways I care for friends and family. Cooking is a tremendous creative outlet for me even though I'm mostly, embarrassingly, a recipe-follower.

I'm eating cake on my birthday, and I hope you do too.

## Inflammation and the Assimilation Node

Because it is home to imbalances in the gastrointestinal system, the Assimilation Node is the most influential node in the matrix. I often refer to the gastrointestinal system as "Grand Central Station." The Assimilation Node includes how we move things from outside our bodies to inside our bodies: digestion and absorption, the respiratory system and the skin. Leaky gut syndrome, the result of intestinal permeability, is a root cause of inflammation. Many physiologic imbalances are the result of inflammatory processes.

Improving intestinal health often involves eliminating foods that are inflammatory for you. Changing what you eat is a simple intervention that stands to improve so much of what ails you. It is simpler than chasing symptoms, popping pills, and dealing with the snowball of side effects from taking multiple medications. Yet changing what you eat can be one of the most challenging things you do. Humans are creatures of habit. Quality food is expensive. Unprocessed food takes time and energy to prepare. Fresh food rots. Twenty-first century living is poorly suited to eating food that comes from the earth. We go too fast. We don't want to take the time, use the energy, or spend the money. We want that Starbucks latte and a muffin to go with it. But good food is less expensive—in terms of time, money, and energy—than being sick.

What we put in
our mouths is **the single
largest variable
within our control**
to affect our health.

———————————

Over 100 trillion microbes live in our gut. They are supposed to be there. These microbes are being studied and linked to specific illnesses and diseases. The microbes exist in balance: too many or too few of any particular microbe can lead to significant physiologic imbalances that result in people feeling quite sick. Improving microbial balance in the gut is the other primary mechanism of healing the gut in addition to modifying what you eat. An overgrowth of gut bacteria that leads to disease is called dysbiosis, which is the root cause of many diseases. Dysbiosis can result from stress, exposure to medication or toxins, or eating inflammatory foods.

I recently saw a woman in her mid-thirties with a history of long-term antibiotic use for cystic acne. She also experienced recurrent sinusitis, diarrhea, infertility, depression, and weight gain. She used Splenda every day in her coffee and drank at least two glasses of wine every night. As an initial intervention, I suggested she eliminate Splenda and reduce her wine consumption. She made no bones about how difficult the latter would be for her. She really liked wine. Food elimination: simple, yet complicated.

## The Digestive Tract

The digestive tract starts in the mouth and ends at the anus. It includes the salivary glands, pancreas, gall bladder, and appendix. The digestive tract:

* breaks down nutrients
* assists with nutrient absorption
* regulates the excretion of water and electrolytes
* eliminates waste and toxins through the stool

For your digestive system to function well, you need normal stomach acidity, adequate levels of digestive enzymes, bile acids, balanced flora, and an intact intestinal lining. The pancreas is responsible for producing essential digestive enzymes and insulin. Insulin is the hormone responsible for blood sugar regulation. Blood sugar stabilization is essential for energy production and hormone balance and is key to preventing inflammation.

The gall bladder stores bile made in the liver. Bile contains bile acids, critical for digestion and absorption of fat and fat-soluble vitamins in the small intestine. Without bile acids, we cannot properly metabolize fat, nor can we absorb fat-soluble vitamins A, D, E, and K. Many waste products are eliminated from the body by secretion into bile and elimination in feces.

The appendix, once deemed nonessential, is now considered a critical component of the immune system. The appendix houses lymphatic tissue and good bacteria that strengthen the immune system. Without your appendix, your immune system is compromised.

Lymphatic tissue lines the gastrointestinal tract. MALT initiates an immune response to specific invaders (antigens) encountered along all mucosal surfaces. MALT can function independently of the systemic immune system, and therefore is an important source of immune system dysregulation. GALT is specific to the gastrointestinal system. MALT and GALT connect the intestines to the immune system through what we eat.

The vagus nerve serves as a two-lane highway between the gut and the brain: The brain talks to the intestines, and the intestines talk to the brain. This highway is the road by which inflammatory substances, like lipopolysaccharides (LPS), travel from a leaky gut to the brain, triggering brain inflammation. Brain inflammation can manifest as foggy thinking, fatigue, memory loss, dementia, and attention deficit disorder.

LPS damages the mitochondria, the energy production centers of cells (see chapter 5, about the Energy Node, for more about the mitochondria). The blood-brain barrier is a network of vessels and tissue comprised of tightly knit cells that keep harmful substances from reaching the brain. Leaky gut leads to a leaky brain because the blood-brain barrier is permeable, just like the lining of the intestines.

## Healing the Gut

IFM developed a program to systematically address gastrointestinal function in five steps. It is called the 5R framework: remove, replace, reinoculate, repair, and rebalance. The goals of this program are to:

- address dietary and lifestyle issues and begin the process of dietary education and change
- normalize digestion and absorption
- normalize the balance of gastrointestinal bacteria
- promote a balanced system of detoxification
- promote gastrointestinal healing

In step one, things negatively affecting the environment of the gastrointestinal tract are **removed**. This includes removing allergenic foods, parasites, dysbiosis, and yeast. Step two involves **replacing** what is missing. Digestive enzymes, hydrochloric acid, and bile salts are added back to the gut. Step three is to **reinoculate**, which involves helping beneficial bacteria flourish through probiotic supplementation or pro- and prebiotic rich foods. Step four is to **repair** the gastrointestinal tract. This includes supplying key nutrients like fish oil and glutamine. And step five is to **rebalance** through lifestyle modification. This is the simplest and hardest step. It may involve long-term elimination of alcohol, ensuring adequate sleep, or refining stress management and coping strategies to reduce the effect of stress on the gut. Lifestyle modifications diminish the likelihood of recurrence.

## The Intricate Web

I first met Daphne more than ten years ago. A forty-five-year-old married woman, she came to Women to Women with a diagnosis of fibromyalgia. I'm sharing her case with you through the Assimilation Node, but many of the nodes were involved. Her story represents how when you pull on one thread in a web, the shape of the whole web changes; when one node in the matrix is addressed, symptoms in the other nodes are affected as well.

Conventional medicine has little to offer people with fibromyalgia other than medication to control symptoms. "Fibromyalgia" is a fancy word that means the body aches. A diagnosis of fibromyalgia does nothing to explain the cause of the body aches. Daphne experienced full-body pain as well as debilitating premenstrual syndrome (PMS) and depression. She also experienced exhaustion, migraines, irritable bowel syndrome, anxiety, and skin flare-ups over the years. When Daphne's fibromyalgia was at its worst, she also experienced stiff joints, excessive burping, and a fullness in her ears.

Our first strategy was to eliminate potentially triggering foods. The primary purpose of food elimination is to decrease inflammation. The process of food elimination and food re-introduction raises your awareness of what you eat and how it makes you feel. The idea that what we eat affects how we feel physically, mentally, and emotionally is novel for many. I've cared for countless women with irritable bowel syndrome and

# The brain talks to the gut,
and the guts talk to the brain.

joint pain. Eliminating artificial sweeteners by removing diet soda often yields significant relief from, if not resolution of, symptoms. No medication necessary. Resolution of symptoms is not always this easily attained, but food elimination is a simple place to start. When Daphne ate ice cream, she experienced muscle pain, joint pain, and migraines. The less ice cream she ate, the better her muscles, joints, and head felt.

I recommend food sensitivity testing less often than I used to. Gluten, grains that cross-react with gluten, and dairy are the most likely food-based inflammatory triggers. When some people with gluten sensitivity eat other grains like rice, millet, or quinoa, their body responds to these other grains as if they ate gluten. If someone presents with irritable bowel syndrome or fibromyalgia, it's unlikely that foods such as blueberries, cinnamon, or cucumbers are the culprit of their pain. Women are, however, prone to over-consuming "healthy" foods like chicken, almonds, and kale. Overconsumption of even otherwise healthy foods can lead to those foods being a source of inflammation.

Daphne was needle-phobic. She did not want to do food sensitivity testing or have any other blood work done. So, in lieu of testing, she opted to eat primarily vegetables and protein.

Early in her journey, removing inflammatory foods from her diet did not completely rebalance Daphne's digestive system. Her symptoms persisted. Daphne and her husband traveled frequently for work. Sometimes, traveling made it difficult for her to eat well. I encouraged Daphne to not skip meals, to increase her dietary protein, and to decrease her carbohydrate intake.

After several years of working together, Daphne did have labs drawn. She got to a point where she wanted data. With the support of a counselor and eye movement desensitization and reprocessing (EMDR), a modality used to treat people with trauma, and a prescription sedative from me, she went to the lab and had testing done for the first time in her adult life.

## ASSIMILATION NODE: CONVENTIONAL LABS

**Comprehensive metabolic panel (CMP).** A blood test that measures glucose levels, electrolyte and fluid balance, and kidney and liver function.

**Complete blood count with differential (CBC with differential).** A blood test used to evaluate overall health and detect a wide range of disorders. The differential evaluates white blood cells, which are elements of the immune system. This can help identify what is taxing the immune system. For example, eosinophil cells become active in the later stages of inflammation. These white blood cells respond to allergic and parasitic disease. One-third of the body's histamine is found in the eosinophilic cell.

**Fasting and two-hour insulin and glucose.** A blood test measuring insulin and glucose levels first thing in the morning before eating and again after consuming a large amount of carbohydrates. Consuming a large amount of carbohydrates challenges the pancreas to make enough insulin to metabolize the carbohydrates. This blood test is the gold standard used to diagnose insulin resistance and type 2 diabetes.

**HgA1c.** A blood test that reflects blood sugar stability over the last three months.

**High-sensitivity C-reactive protein (hs-CRP).** A blood test for markers of systemic inflammation. Hs-CRP is a surrogate marker for interleukins, proteins made by white blood cells that regulate immune responses. Hs-CRP screens for infections and inflammatory diseases. It does not diagnose a specific disease.

**Vitamin D3.** A blood test measuring vitamin D3 levels in the body. Two forms of vitamin D are important for nutrition:

D2 and D3. Vitamin D2 mainly comes from fortified foods like breakfast cereals, milk, and other dairy items. Vitamin D3 is made by your body when you are exposed to sunlight. It is also found in some foods, including eggs and fatty fish such as salmon, tuna, and mackerel. Vitamin D is essential for healthy bones and teeth.

## ASSIMILATION NODE: FUNCTIONAL LABS

**Comprehensive Nutritional Evaluation.** A blood and urine test used to evaluate the functional need for antioxidants, B vitamins, minerals, essential fatty acids, amino acids, digestive support, and other select nutrients. The test also screens for heavy metal toxicity and markers of dysbiosis and candida. Results provide a personalized vitamin and amino acid prescription.

**Food sensitivity testing.** Blood tests measuring IgG immunoglobulin levels in response to specific food proteins. True food allergies, like anaphylaxis from eating peanuts, are determined by measuring IgE levels.

**Hydrogen breath test.** A breath test to measure hydrogen and methane, which can be detected through the breath after consuming a specific drink. Elevated levels are indicative of small intestinal bacterial overgrowth (SIBO). This test is available through conventional and functional laboratories. Insurance may cover the cost of the test when processed through a conventional laboratory. The advantage of testing through a functional lab is that the test can be completed at home.

**Intestinal permeability test.** A urinary test that measures the excretion of sugars and their ratio as a basis for measuring intestinal permeability.

**Stool testing.** A one-day stool collection, done at home, measuring gastrointestinal microbiota DNA. The test detects parasites, bacteria, fungi, and more. It measures indicators of digestion, absorption, inflammation, and immune function.

## Emotional Work

Daphne's journey toward wholeness included deep emotional work related to childhood trauma. Nine years into our work together, Daphne began to have skin flare-ups. Her first flare occurred while she was traveling out of state for work. She sent me photographs of bright red skin behind her ears, under her breasts, and down her abdomen and legs. Food elimination, supplements, and topical steroids did not improve her skin; the only intervention that helped was emotional healing. Through introspection, self-observation, and work with a therapist, she learned to connect feelings of neglect with her skin flare-ups.

Many months later, Daphne experienced an increase in anxiety, which she attributed to a pending move. Her anxiety was so severe that she was unable to be alone at home or to drive. She was having more migraines. The sense of fullness in her ears persisted.

She did, however, have less muscle pain. Daphne and her husband had embraced eating local, non-processed, anti-inflammatory foods no matter where they were, including while they traveled. They ate mostly protein and vegetables. They loved finding local farmer's markets, preparing and consuming beautiful food, the bounty unique to each season, and the creative expression of cooking. They exemplified food-first medicine living.

## ASSIMILATION NODE: LIFESTYLE MODIFICATIONS

**Eliminate all artificial sweeteners.** This is the only "food" to *never* eat. Artificial sweeteners are *not food*. They are chemicals, proven to cause cancer in laboratory animals. Because artificial sweeteners are not recognized by the body as food, the body responds to them as toxins. The inflammation caused by the consumption of artificial sweeteners is often the root cause, or a significant part of the root cause, of chronic fatigue syndrome, irritable bowel syndrome, and fibromyalgia. Choose local honey or maple syrup instead. Not only are they unprocessed and sweet, but they are also rich in beneficial prebiotics.

**Eat food from the earth.** Foods that can be hunted or gathered are the best for us. Food from the earth is not packaged or processed. It is nutrient dense and has a short shelf life. Look to local farmers and farmers markets for fresh, seasonal food. The quicker food gets from the farm to the table, the more nutrient dense it is. Eat foods in season—asparagus and rhubarb in the spring, zucchini and tomatoes in the summer, apples and acorn squash in the fall, potatoes and other root vegetables in the winter. Eating greens in the winter is a luxury of twenty-first century living! Consider reserving foods such as corn and summer squash for the summertime. The benefits of eating local food, supporting local farms, and participating in your community extend beyond physical health.

**Eat the rainbow.** Eating foods of varying color every day supports all the nodes. Foods rich in color have high levels of antioxidants. The more colorful the foods you consume, the more antioxidants you get. Foods with different colors are phytonutrient rich in different ways. Phytonutrient diversity is key to optimal health. Eating the same foods every day limits nutrient availability. Ask yourself, have I eaten red foods today? orange? yellow? green? For blue foods, think blueberries, blue potatoes, and elderberries; for purple, think purple kale, eggplant, and purple cabbage.

**Eat different things from day to day.** Eating the same thing every day significantly limits the phytonutrient diversity of your diet. You have to eat a variety of foods to get a variety of nutrients. Plan at least four different go-to breakfasts, lunches, and dinners that you rotate eating regularly. Over-consuming a specific food, even a food considered healthy, can result in that food triggering an inflammatory response. Eat a variety of nuts, not just almonds. Use a variety of oils, mostly olive and coconut, but not processed oils like canola. Eat a variety of vegetables, fruits, and proteins.

**Plan a menu.** Menu planning helps diversify what you eat. Having a roster of a few simple meals you can prepare easily, such as black bean burrito bowls and stir-fries, when plans change, the day gets away from you, or your energy level is low, is critical. It is easier to make good food choices if good food is on hand.

Try this method: Review the days of the week and your evening commitments to identify who will be home, who will be busy, who will likely cook, and when having leftovers might reduce the stress of an evening. Note the proteins— one night is beef, one night is fish, one night is vegetarian, one night is chicken, and so forth. Consider the season— more soups and stews in the winter, more salads and grilling in the summer. Consult cookbooks, apps, and websites for inspiring recipes. The *New York Times* has a blog that nods to the season and provides a menu for the week: *What to Cook This Week* is a reasonable place to start. Then, make a grocery list and go shopping. Double or triple the quantity of recipes so there are leftovers for other dinners or lunches during the week, or meals in the coming week (hello, freezer!).

If you love cooking, cookbooks, and finding new recipes, this approach may be more appealing than if you are not inclined to cook. But even if the latter is true for you, seek options that ensure you get a variety of phytonutrient sources (for example, healthy food delivery services or preprepared food made of whole foods—check the ingredients lists!).

## Eating for the Assimilation Node

Daphne's pain diminished over time in response to her dietary changes and being treated for systemic yeast. Eliminating sugar and following an Anti-Candida Food Plan significantly improved her symptoms.

Systemic yeast, systemic candida, chronic yeast, yeast overgrowth, or candida overgrowth are interchangeable terms used to describe the overgrowth of yeast in the intestines. Yeast overgrowth is a diagnosis frequently dismissed by conventional medical practitioners unless someone is severely immunocompromised, for example, a person with the human immunodeficiency virus (HIV) or undergoing cancer treatment. For non-conventional practitioners, yeast overgrowth is a relatively common diagnosis, and the condition responds well to nutritional and botanical intervention.

Yeast is part of our normal bacterial flora and, in and of itself, is not problematic. It is part of the balance in our microbiome. Yeast becomes problematic when it proliferates and overgrows. Sugar cravings, constipation, itching—particularly around the rectum or in the ears—depression, muscle pain, or recurrent sinusitis are symptoms suggesting a yeast overgrowth.

When women say, "I can't eat just one cookie. If I eat one, I'm eating the entire package," I think yeast overgrowth. Women with a family history of alcoholism often have this all-or-nothing relationship with sugar. Alcohol is essentially sugar, so dietary consumption of sugar can trigger the same addictive pathways in the brain.

Yeast overgrowth does not always present as a vaginal yeast infection, although it can and does. Yeast overgrowth points to the importance of balance in the body: some yeast, essential; too much yeast, a problem. A body in balance, for the most part, can handle small amounts of anything—alcohol, sugar, grains. Women who experience yeast overgrowth seem to have a lower threshold of tolerance and an increased susceptibility for recurrence; they have less "wiggle room," by which I mean that after treatment and resolution and the resumption of a normal diet, some women's threshold for recurrence seems lower than that of women who have never experienced yeast overgrowth.

The holiday season can pose a challenge when food elimination is the primary treatment. Food elimination can be a source of stress and social isolation. Some women are so invested in feeling better that the holidays are not a deterrent for them. Gluten, dairy, and sugar crept back into Daphne's diet during the holidays. She experienced increased fatigue, anxiety, and pain. She resumed eating gluten-free and dairy-free, took up the Anti-Candida Food Plan again, and restarted treatment for yeast overgrowth.

Daphne attributed the unrelenting pain of her fibromyalgia, primarily in her hamstrings and feet, to eating more carbohydrates. Things were worse for her, physically and emotionally, in the winter. She addressed this by increasing her vitamin D3 and fish oil supplementation as well as adding a shake rich in the anti-inflammatory herbs turmeric and rosemary leaf.

Daphne's combination of eating well and nutrient repletion resulted in less anxiety. She had fewer headaches, less pain and fullness in her ears, good energy, and good sleep. When yeast flared, joint pain and sinus congestion flared too. She learned

Because we are biochemically unique, **the "right" way to eat is different for each of us.**

---

that when she flared, she could look at what she'd been eating, find the trigger, and eliminate it. I knew we'd made significant progress when she said, "It doesn't hurt to be hugged anymore."

## ASSIMILATION NODE: NUTRITION INTERVENTIONS

**Consume more vegetables.** Vegetables are rich in soluble fiber, which may ensure the formation of normal stool and normal travel time of stool through the colon. Vegetables also provide insoluble fiber and resistant starch from which organisms in the microbiota make short-chain fatty acids (SCFAS). SCFAS include acetate, propionate, and butyrate. SCFAS are used by enterocytes, cells lining the intestine, or are transported across the gut tissue into the bloodstream, where they affect metabolism, inflammation, and the development of disease.

**Eat fermented foods.** Fermented foods are rich in pre- and probiotics, strengthening the immune system and helping balance the gut microbiome. Fermented foods include sauerkraut, kimchi, kombucha, yogurt, and kefir. Fermented foods may be contraindicated for people with yeast overgrowth or dairy sensitivity; otherwise, incorporating these foods into your diet daily can be beneficial.

**Eat apples.** Apples have over one hundred million bacteria that populate our microbiome. Apples are rich in both pre- and probiotics, pectin, minerals, soluble and insoluble fiber, and polyphenols like quercetin. Apples are high in FODMAPS (fermentable oligosaccharides, disaccharides, monosaccharides, and polyols), simple sugars that are not easily absorbed and quickly ferment in the gut, and are contraindicated for people following a low-FODMAP diet.

**Consume bone broth.** Bone broth is rich in minerals, collagen, and amino acids. It supports connective tissue, joints, gut healing, muscle building, and mood.

**Take coconut, in all its forms.** Coconut is a medium-chain triglyceride and is absorbed directly by the small intestine. The body rapidly uptakes coconut for energy. Coconut is high in manganese, which is good for bones and the metabolism of carbohydrates and protein; is rich in antioxidants; and is made of lauric acid, which has antimicrobial and anti-inflammatory effects.

## Therapeutic food plans

Numerous therapeutic food plans facilitate healing the Assimilation Node, depending on an individual's imbalance. In fact, there are so many therapeutic food plans it can be difficult to identify which one is best for a person given their symptoms. Therapeutic food plans are intended to be nutritional interventions. *They are not intended to be a lifestyle.* Staying on therapeutic food plans over the long term can result in untoward health effects. Work with a seasoned practitioner to identify which plan is best for you. The following is a mere overview of therapeutic food plans. Entire books have been written about each of them. I've included a few in the resources section at the end of this book for your reference.

**Autoimmune Protocol.** A plan aimed to reduce inflammation and relieve symptoms of autoimmune disorders. It is an extension of the Paleo diet, otherwise known as "the caveman" diet. It includes vegetables, except nightshades; seafood; fermented foods; lean meats and liver; small amounts of fruit; and oils.

**Core Food Plan.** Developed by IFM, a therapeutic food plan that may benefit women who are transitioning from a Standard American Diet (SAD) to more nutritious eating. The Core Food Plan is suitable to adapt for the long term. It is based on the Mediterranean diet and focuses on whole foods, promotes clean and organic foods, ensures adequate intake of protein, balances quality fats, is high in fiber and low in simple sugars, and promotes phytonutrient diversity.

**Elimination Diet.** A three-week nutrition intervention that promotes body awareness of food and identifies food triggers. It reduces inflammation, supports a healthy microbiome, is dairy- and gluten-free, reduces toxic burden, and has no calorie restriction.

**Gut and Psychology Syndrome Diet (GAPS).** A specific carbohydrate diet (SCD, see below), with a few modifications: fewer beans, no baking soda, no store-bought juice. Cultured vegetables are emphasized in place of yogurt. The GAPS diet incorporates the nutritional guidelines of the Weston A. Price Foundation.

**Low-FODMAP (fermentable oligosaccharides, disaccharides, monosaccharides, and polyols).** An eating plan that eliminates foods comprised of short-chain carbohydrates resistant to digestion. Instead of being absorbed into the bloodstream, these carbohydrates collect at the end of the intestines, where gut bacteria use them for fuel, producing hydrogen gas. This gas can cause intestinal distress in sensitive individuals. Common FODMAPs are fructose, including fruit sugar; lactose, found in dairy; fructans, found in many grains; galactans, found in legumes; and polyols, which are sugar alcohols like xylitol.

**SIBO Diet.** A therapeutic nutrition plan combining SCD and low-FODMAP, used to treat small intestinal bacterial overgrowth (SIBO).

**Specific Carbohydrate Diet (SCD).** A grain-free food plan, low in sugar and lactose, initially developed to treat celiac disease. The SCD is used to treat irritable bowel syndrome.

## Supplements

**Bile acid replacements.** Nausea after eating fatty food and tan colored stools that float are symptoms of poor fat metabolism. Bile acids are essential for digesting fat and absorbing fat-soluble vitamins A, D, E, and K. Bile acid replacement is essential for people who do not have a gall bladder.

**Digestive enzymes.** Essential for digesting fats, carbohydrates, and proteins, digestive enzymes are depleted by stress, processed food, and antibiotics. As a supplement, they are taken with the major meals of the day. Bitters can be used to stimulate digestive enzyme production in lieu of, or in addition to, supplementation.

**Hydrochloric acid (HCL).** Low HCL, or hypochlorhydria, a deficiency of stomach acid, is a common cause of heartburn and reflux. Over-the-counter antacids like TUMS and Pepcid compound hypochlorhydria. HCL cleaves vitamin B12, an essential B vitamin, from meat. Vegetarians benefit from supplementing with B12. HCL production declines with age.

**L-glutamine.** An amino acid that facilitates healing of the gap junctions in the small intestine, repairing leaky gut.

**Probiotics.** Microorganisms that restore beneficial bacteria in the gut, probiotics are essential for microbial balance. They reinforce the immune system. Specific strains of probiotics are used to treat specific symptoms.

## Peeling the Onion
. . . . . . . . . . . . . . . . . . .

My husband once asked me, "Do you recommend *everyone* not eat gluten?" Embedded in his question is a healthy skepticism of dietary trends. I am skeptical too. I have met women who cured themselves of cancer through a macrobiotic diet, and I have met women who have been hospitalized for nutrient deficiency as the result of eating a macrobiotic diet. Similarly, I have met women who feel energized and strong after the Whole 30 diet and women who were insatiably hungry and light-headed on the Whole 30. *There is no one-size-fits-all "diet."* Because we are biochemically unique, the "right" way to eat is different for each of us. I was a vegetarian for many years, and I've never been more fatigued or weighed more in my life, other than when I was pregnant. Alternately, when I eat Paleo, I find myself insatiably hungry. I feel best when I eat mostly vegetables, small amounts of high-quality animal protein, lots of nuts and seeds, and small amounts of complex carbohydrates.

We tend to subscribe to other people's ideas about what is good for us to eat. We distrust our lived experience about what we know to be true about our bodies. Surviving trauma, of whatever variety, makes us experts at living disconnected from our physical bodies. The seventy-two-billion-dollar weight-loss industry fuels and preys on our distrust of ourselves. Connecting what we put in our mouths with our lived experience of how it makes us feel is a challenge.

Daphne's story is good example of how getting well is rarely a linear process. It is like peeling an onion—layers and layers of imbalance have to be restored for wellness to emerge. Food elimination is not intended to be forever, except when there is a true food allergy. Food allergies are identified through IgE testing or the lived experience of hives or anaphylaxis in response to eating an allergenic food. My goal when working with women is to help the gut heal so that small amounts of any food can be tolerated. I remind women that a particular food is not the problem, the problem is our physiologic response to it, which is largely determined by what is going on in our gut.

# 8

# The Real Deal with Detox

· · · · · · · · · · · · · · · · ·

## BIOTRANSFORMATION AND ELIMINATION NODE:
### TOXICITY, DETOXIFICATION

DETOXIFICATION IS *a complicated metabolic process influenced by your genes, nutrition, and environment. Adequate detoxification is essential to life: to at least survive, if not thrive, you have to be able to manage pesticide exposure from your food, chemicals in your objects of daily living, and environmental toxins. Your liver is the hub of detoxification in your body. Alcohol use and consumption of over-the-counter medications add to its burden. Women with imbalances in this node often present with sensitivities to medications, cleaning products, perfumes, and the like. They may also have fibroids, endometriosis, infertility, or breast cancer.*

WHEN I first started clinical practice, I didn't even know "detoxing" was "a thing." I'd heard of "cleanses" but had never been compelled to do one. The closest I'd come was eliminating sugar on a yoga retreat. A friend in college did multiple "detoxes," and at the time, I thought she was unhinged. I was first introduced to the physiology of detoxification through impaired hormone detoxification as a root cause of hormone imbalance.

If you take care of women long enough and actually listen to them, eventually the topic of "doing a detox" comes up, typically as a weight-loss strategy. Detoxing has grown in popularity over the decades I've cared for women. I am amazed by the contortions people are willing to put themselves through to detox. If it's true that we store trauma in our cells and toxins are stored in fat cells, then I don't think we can ever be entirely "clean." I, myself, am more of a slow-and-steady-forward kind of gal than a wham-bam, clear-the-deck kind of gal. But I take care of all kinds of women.

Women with detoxification issues are some of the sickest I care for. Life on Earth is dangerous for them; they never know which bug bite, which cleaning product, or which food exposure might throw them into a state that takes an unforeseeable amount of time to recover from. Sometimes a severe allergic reaction requires epinephrine or a trip to the emergency room; sometimes there is pain or gastrointestinal distress, hives, or brain fog. An overburdened body is unpredictable. I often feel like I'm out of my league caring for these women because their health histories are typically quite complex. They frequently end up in my office because conventional medical practitioners simply do not know how to care for them.

Fear often accompanies such women and their symptoms. How much fear is part of the *cause of* the problem as opposed to how much fear is a healthy *response to* the problem is impossible to untangle. Feeling fearful is a healthy response when your health—or life—is threatened. Either way, you have to contend with fear because fear, in and of itself, has its own bearing on your health.

I've grown to appreciate the tremendous work our livers do, quietly filtering the toxins we encounter every day, keeping us well. I've grown to appreciate how human behavior adds to the burden on our livers, whether because we take prescription or over-the-counter medication, drink alcohol, eat processed food, clean with chemicals, or live in a city.

Our genes are the wild card influencing the extent to and efficiency with which we can detoxify. Without the right genes, the multistep process of detoxification is compromised and may require support.

In addition to physical detoxification, there is emotional detoxification to consider as well. Emotionally difficult relationships, unsatisfying work, or too much screen time all have ill effects on your health. Your cells are bathed not only in chemical information by way of what you ingest and your physical environment but also in the energetics of your thoughts.

Detox support calls us to be our witchiest selves—drinking tea; taking a bath; sweating in a sauna, on a run, or in a yoga class; getting off our devices; foraging for food; moving in ways that may appear unacceptable; screaming or crying; pooping; grounding ourselves with our bare feet against the earth. I am partial to a lifestyle that supports detoxification, as opposed to "doing a detox," but there's no right way, nor is there one way.

## The Science of Biotransformation and Elimination

Many women come to the clinic wanting to "detox," thinking of detoxing as a shortcut to wellness and weight loss. Detoxification is a complex metabolic process involving multiple enzymes and multiple steps. Detoxification requires having enough of the right vitamins and minerals on board to support the process, and a healthy gut. The liver dumps to the gut, so when the microbiome of the gut is not balanced, detoxification can make us feel worse, not better. A few days of drinking lemon juice and cayenne in water is not a cure-all. Detoxification requires working enzyme systems, nutrient support, sufficient calories, and peeing, pooping, and sweating.

Every body is different. The amount of toxic exposure one person can withstand while maintaining health differs from another. We are biochemically unique. Our ability to detoxify is influenced by:

- genes
- diet
- gastrointestinal health
- nutritional status
- stress levels
- exposure to toxins

Some pregnant women smoke cigarettes, eat Ho Hos, and have perfectly healthy babies. Other pregnant women eat lots of vegetables, exercise regularly, and do not have healthy babies. Why? Because every body endures a different toxic load and every body's ability to detoxify is different. I took care of a woman who did not drive her car on the highway in the city. The air was so polluted that even when filtered through her car, it triggered her to vomit. Her toxic load and body burden, the amount of toxic chemicals in her system, were high.

Weight is not a calorie in, calorie out equation. Most of us do not lose weight by eating less and exercising more. Weight is generally a symptom of an underlying physiologic imbalance. A woman's weight typically normalizes when the physiologic balance is restored through working the nodes of the matrix. A supported detoxification program may be helpful.

Completely avoiding toxic exposure and toxins in our lives is impossible. I've witnessed too many women experience fear and subsequent isolation as the result of adopting extreme measures, although sometimes extreme measures are necessary. I've seen women quit jobs, move houses, and leave relationships all in an effort to reduce their toxic exposure—sometimes with fantastic results. You *do* want to minimize your exposure to toxins and optimize your detoxification processes. Avoid what feels reasonable to avoid, with the operative word being "reasonable."

## Toxin Elimination

Toxins go through a three-step process in the liver that readies them for elimination.

**Phase I** of detoxification, known as oxidation, involves enzymes neutralizing substances such as caffeine, nicotine, and alcohol and converting chemicals into intermediate substances for further processing and elimination. This process can result in oxidative stress and an excess of free radicals, those unstable molecules that damage other molecules. If toxic intermediates build up in the body, they can damage DNA and proteins. Toxic intermediates are often more toxic than the original compounds.

Our genetic makeup affects how this process works and people's ability to detoxify. Essential nutrients to support Phase I of detoxification include B vitamins (including folic acid), vitamin E, vitamin C, magnesium, and zinc.

**Phase II** of detoxification, also known as conjugation, neutralizes those Phase I intermediates and transforms them into compounds that can be eliminated from the body. In Phase II, various enzymes protect us from getting cancer. When these enzymes are not working well, a person is at increased risk of

# An overburdened body **is unpredictable.**

---

developing cancer. Nutrients that support Phase II detoxification include amino acids (glutamine, glycine, taurine, and cysteine) and sulphate phytochemicals found in cruciferous vegetables. A process called methylation also occurs in Phase II. Methylation turns genes on and off. Methylation also regulates neurotransmitters, brain function, mood, energy, and hormone levels. Homocysteine is an amino acid and a product of methylation. Elevated homocysteine levels indicate a vitamin B6, vitamin B12, or folate deficiency, often the result of an inability to convert folate to a usable form. The inability to convert folate to its active form can lead to an increased risk of heart disease and atherosclerosis. Low levels of homocysteine are indicative of a slow methylation cycle and low levels of glutathione, the master antioxidant in the body.

**Phase III** of detoxification, also known as elimination, involves the transport of water-soluble intermediary compounds like glutathione and sulfate out of cells and into the bile in the liver for elimination. Phase III transporters are proteins called ATP-binding cassette (ABC) transporters. ABC transporters require chemical energy in the form of adenosine triphosphate (ATP, cellular energy) to pump toxins through cell membranes, out of the cells.

Bile is critical for moving toxins out of the liver and into the intestines. Impaired bile production because of the absence of a gall bladder can compromise a person's ability to detoxify. Impaired bile flow, or cholestasis, resulting from dysfunction within the liver or blockage of the bile duct, can result in a build-up of liver toxins. In the kidneys and intestines, Phase III transporters remove toxins from the blood for excretion through urine and stool.

When our bodies can't clear toxins as quickly as they accumulate, our immune system is activated. The accumulation of toxins signals danger to the immune system. This is described by immunologists as "not being able to clear the debris field." An accumulation of toxins in the body, or a cluttered debris field, leads to "loss of tolerance." Loss of tolerance is when people react to things such as food and environmental exposures that previously did not adversely affect them. The interaction between inflammation and immune system signaling is expanded on in the Defense and Repair Node chapter (chapter 10).

## When a Health Crisis Leads to Transformation

Suzanne is fair-skinned and petite. She speaks quietly and with conviction. She lives a relatively alternative lifestyle in a rural part of Maine. We have worked together for more than a decade, and I've witnessed her transition from an administrator to a body-based therapist. Her transition was one of necessity: Her health required her to control her work schedule. She has survived multiple healing crises, including, early in our acquaintance, a hospitalization that saved her life. She has physically, emotionally, and spiritually transformed in response to her healing crises.

Suzanne was one of the sickest women I encountered while working at Women to Women. She traveled hours to come to the clinic and needed someone to drive her. In her forties and married, she was barely able to stand, emaciated, and pale. She was struggling to keep her job.

She'd had a hysterectomy and a long history of gut issues. Her most recent hospitalization was the result of gluten toxicity. Suzanne was unable to go grocery shopping because the supermarket made her feel sick, especially the aisle with household cleaners. She exhibited symptoms of multiple chemical sensitivity (MCS). People with MCS have low or no tolerance to fragrance, chemicals of any kind, and sometimes their environment.

Eventually, she opted to do a blood test that screened for exposure to toxins like BPA (bisphenol A), parabens, and heavy metals.

## BIOTRANSFORMATION AND
## ELIMINATION NODE: CONVENTIONAL LABS

**Complete blood count (CBC).** A blood test used to evaluate overall health and detect a wide range of disorders including anemia, infection, and leukemia.

**Comprehensive metabolic panel (CMP).** A blood test that measures glucose levels, electrolyte and fluid balance, and kidney and liver function.

**Homocysteine.** A blood test that measures this amino acid in the blood. Vitamins B6, B12, and folate are necessary to metabolize homocysteine, such that increased levels of the amino acid may be a sign of deficiency in those vitamins. Homocysteine is also used as a systemic inflammation marker.

**High-sensitivity C-reactive protein (hs-CRP).** A high-sensitivity blood test for a marker of systemic inflammation. Hs-CRP is a surrogate marker for interleukins, proteins made by white blood cells that regulate immune responses. Hs-CRP screens for infections and inflammatory diseases. This test does not diagnose a specific disease.

**Methylenetetrahydrofolate reductase (MTHFR).** A blood test can detect the two most common mutations of the MTHFR gene, which contain the code to produce the MTHFR enzyme. The enzyme is critical for metabolizing one form of B vitamin, folate, into another.

## BIOTRANSFORMATION AND
## ELIMINATION NODE: FUNCTIONAL LABS

**Chemical immune reactivity screen.** This blood test identifies environmental triggers for people with impaired biotransformation. Results inform lifestyle decisions on how to reduce exposure to them.

**Comprehensive Nutritional Evaluation.** A blood and urine test used to evaluate the functional need for antioxidants, B vitamins, minerals, essential fatty acids, amino acids, digestive support, and other select nutrients. The test also screens for heavy metal toxicity and measures micronutrients essential for optimal ATP production.

**Genomic testing.** A sample of cells from the cheek used to identify single nucleotide polymorphisms (SNPs) associated with increased risk of impaired detoxification capacity, either related to environmental toxins or hormone metabolism. Genetic expression is significantly influenced by the environment in which genes live.

**Methylation panel.** Methylation metabolites are measured in plasma, and genetic single nucleotide polymorphisms (SNPs) are analyzed via a cheek swab. Offers insight into the nutrients and genes that regulate the methylation pathway.

**Mycotoxin panel.** A urine test used to assess for mycotoxins (substances produced by a variety of molds).

**Stool testing.** A one-day stool collection, done at home, measuring gastrointestinal microbiota DNA. The test detects parasites, bacteria, fungi, and more. It measures indicators of digestion, absorption, inflammation, and immune function.

## Supporting Biotransformation and Elimination

After being hospitalized, Suzanne eliminated gluten, but her anxiety and fatigue were so severe that she still could not grocery shop. It remained unclear whether other dietary triggers perpetuated the inflammation, or the damage to her tissues from gluten toxicity were so severe that it was taking a long time to heal, or her detoxification pathways were still compromised, or all of the above.

To reduce the physiologic burden of inflammation on her body, Suzanne looked to lifestyle factors she could modulate to reduce stress. Changing careers enabled her to control her workflow and schedule. She could work the number of days a week and see the number of clients a day that she felt able to. She could schedule rest. She had more time for her own daily practice and caring for her aging mother. She followed a low-FODMAP diet but did not tolerate probiotics or digestive enzymes. She added zinc, vitamin C, and B vitamins. She considered a trial of amino acid supplementation. For a time, Suzanne took antianxiety medication every day. She tried hormone therapy to see if hormone support would help. It did not.

Eventually, she tolerated scented shampoo and going into large stores to shop. These were significant indications of improvement, even though her anxiety and fatigue persisted. She added B12 injections. She increased her vitamin D supplementation. She integrated going to a sauna and sweating daily.

### BIOTRANSFORMATION AND ELIMINATION NODE: LIFESTYLE MODIFICATIONS

**Eat organic and non-GMO.** Eating organic and non-GMO food ensures that the food eaten is nutrient dense and reduces exposure to pesticides. Washing fruits and vegetables further decreases pesticide exposure. Refer to the Environmental Working Groups Clean Fifteen and Dirty Dozen for guidance on which foods are important to buy organic.

**Decrease alcohol consumption.** Research shows health benefits from consuming four ounces of red wine a day. Red wine is a rich source of the phytonutrient resveratrol, a potent anti-inflammatory. Drinking more than four ounces, and even as little as four ounces for some people, increases the toxic burden to the liver. Many women in perimenopause and menopause are unable to tolerate drinking alcohol because it either disrupts sleep, triggers headaches, or contributes to weight gain. Eliminating alcohol overconsumption is the easiest way to slash and burn toxic exposure, not to mention excess carbohydrate consumption. Exposure to toxins in air, food, and water is difficult to control, but we can control our exposure to alcohol.

**Use non-chemical cleaning products.** Using chemical-free cleaning products reduces our individual and environmental exposure to toxins. Most household cleaning can be done using a vinegar and water solution, or a vinegar, water, and dish soap solution. Baking soda is an effective abrasive cleaner.

**Use simple personal care products.** Using unscented shampoo, paraben-free cream, natural deodorant, and baking-soda based toothpaste reduces your exposure to chemicals. Zinc oxide is an effective non-chemical sunscreen.

**Sweat.** Sweat is another key mechanism by which we eliminate toxins, like hormone metabolites, from our bodies. Aerobic exercise, hot yoga, Epsom salt and baking soda baths, and saunas all promote sweating.

**You have to contend with fear** because fear, in and of itself, has its own bearing on your health.

———————————

**Reduce the use of non-steroidal anti-inflammatory medications.** Liberal use of over-the-counter medications burdens our livers significantly. Use non-steroidal anti-inflammatory medications, like aspirin, ibuprofen, and naproxen, judiciously.

**Hydrate.** Adequate hydration supports stool formation and urine production, two primary pathways of elimination. To approximate how much water you need in a day, divide your weight by half and drink that many ounces. For example, if you weigh 140 pounds, drink 70 ounces of water a day. Or, observe the color of your urine when you void. Urine appears clear, like water, when hydration is adequate.

**Decrease exposure to plastic.** Plastic is a significant environmental toxin, not only for humans but also for animals and the planet. We drink from it, eat from it, wear it, and even sleep on it. Use a glass water bottle and glass food storage containers. Wear natural fiber clothing as much as possible.

## Supporting Detoxification

Suzanne added the supplement glutathione, the master antioxidant in the body. With that addition, she experienced a reduction in, if not complete resolution of, anxiety. She added prebiotics, not probiotics, because probiotics made her feel sick. She added l-glutamine to facilitate the healing of her intestinal lining.

Her fatigue was persistent and debilitating, so she tested her adrenal gland function, which was low. Suzanne started an adrenal glandular supplement and added topical pregnenolone, which she tolerated better than estrogen and progesterone.

Anxiety and fatigue waxed and waned depending on her food and chemical exposure. She wanted to decrease her toxic exposure to decrease her overall toxic load, ultimately decreasing her body burden of toxins. Suzanne limited her diet to mostly protein, fruits, and vegetables. She used a vinegar solution for household cleaning and turned to all-natural personal care products. We struggled to identify where her toxic exposure was coming from.

We wondered about her genes and the efficiency of her detoxification pathways, so she did some genomic testing. In response to her test results, I encouraged her to increase her glutathione and add additional detoxification support including CoQ10, alpha-lipoic acid, n-acetylcysteine, hot yoga, and infrared sauna sessions.

## BIOTRANSFORMATION AND ELIMINATION NODE: NUTRITION INTERVENTIONS

**Try the Detox Food Plan.** A therapeutic food plan developed by IFM to support detoxification pathways. The goal of the detox food plan is to reduce food triggers, support liver function, provide the body with a diverse array of phytonutrients, encourage healthy elimination of toxins, and balance hormone metabolism. The Detox Food Plan focuses on long-term nutritional support of the major body systems involved with detoxification including the gut, liver, and kidneys. It strongly emphasizes eating nutrient-dense food for life, reducing food contact with contaminating elements, and eating organic foods when possible.

**Drink green tea.** Green tea provides a rich supply of catechins, potent antioxidants that balance detoxification pathways. The most significant catechin in green tea is epigallocatechin gallate (EGCG), which is associated with a decreased risk of cancer. Citrus amplifies the effects of EGCG, so consuming them together is ideal.

**Eat flax meal.** Flax meal is a rich source of lignan, a fiber-like compound that helps demolish harmful forms of estrogen and promotes stool formation.

**Avoid grapefruit.** Its primary flavonoid, naringenin, inhibits CYP activity (enzymes that help detoxification), inhibiting Phase I detoxification.

**Drink milk thistle tea.** Silymarin is a derivative of milk thistle and acts as an antioxidant. Antioxidants lower oxidative stress in the liver, thereby conserving cellular glutathione.

## Supplements

**Calcium D-glucarate.** A chemical similar to naturally occurring glucaric acid, which is found in the body as well as in fruits and vegetables. Calcium D-glucarate combines glucaric acid with calcium. It supports the body's defense against toxins and excess steroid hormones.

**D-limonene.** A compound found in citrus peel, D-limonene induces Phase I and Phase II enzymes and, therefore, has anti-carcinogenic properties.

**Glutathione.** The key antioxidant that protects the body from intermediary toxins. It provides direct chemical neutralization of free radicals, is a cofactor of several antioxidant enzymes, regenerates vitamins C and E, neutralizes free radicals produced by Phase I detoxification, is one of seven Phase II reactions that makes Phase I intermediates water soluble for excretion by the kidneys, transports mercury out of the cells and brain, regulates cellular proliferation and apoptosis, and is vital to mitochondrial function.

**N-acetyl cysteine (NAC).** The supplement form of cysteine, which provides sulfur for glutathione production, replenishing glutathione stores, thereby reducing oxidative stress. It is used in hospitals to treat Tylenol toxicity.

**Resveratrol.** A potent antiviral and anti-inflammatory nutrient. The phytonutrient present in red wine, resveratrol provides cardioprotective, chemoprotective, and anti-inflammatory benefits. Resveratrol improves vascular function, extends the lifespan, has anti-aging effects, opposes the effects of high-calorie diets, mimics the effects of calorie restriction, and improves cellular function. Resveratrol provides protection against chemical, cholestatic, and alcohol injury to the liver. It decreases liver fibrosis and steatosis.

**Sulforaphane.** A sulfur-rich compound found in cruciferous vegetables such as broccoli and bok choy. Sulforaphane stimulates the production of Phase II detoxification enzymes. Supplementing with sulforaphane can increase the production of protective enzymes.

**Turmeric.** A bright yellow-orange root often ground into spice. The color of turmeric comes mainly from fat-soluble, polyphenolic pigments known as curcuminoids. Curcumin prevents liver injury by modulating Phase I and Phase II liver enzymes and functions as a potent antioxidant.

## Incorporating Detox

One year later, Suzanne returned to the clinic for her annual exam and was feeling pretty good. Vitamin B12 injections reduced her anxiety notably. She was completely and strictly gluten- and dairy-free, and her stomach felt good as long as she was "careful." She had even gained a little weight. She was sleeping well, walking daily, and doing yoga.

Suzanne continued to heal, albeit slowly, until recently. It had been difficult for her to eat in restaurants because she reacted to trace amounts of gluten. She limited her dairy. She gained five pounds in a year. She continued with weekly B12 injections and is certain supplementing with glutathione is what enabled her to return to grocery shopping. She has experienced a significant setback she attributes to receiving a COVID vaccine. She is now working through mold toxicity; mast cell activation syndrome, a condition that causes the mast cells of the immune system to release large amounts of chemicals into the body, causing allergic reactions and a variety of other symptoms; and limbic and vagal nerve dysfunction.

Regularly consuming broccoli, milk thistle tea, green tea, and berries will support your liver and the Biotransformation and Elimination Node, as may supplementing with glutathione or NAC, sweating, and having daily bowel movements. Supporting liver function optimizes the biotransformation and elimination of toxins and, ultimately, your health.

# 9

# What Goes Around

. . . . . . . . . . . . . . . . . . .

*TRANSPORT NODE:*
*CARDIOVASCULAR SYSTEM,*
*LYMPHATIC SYSTEM*

YOU MOVE *a lot of things around your body—oxygen,*

*nutrients, hormones, electrons, and genetic material.*

*When things aren't moving well, your health can go hay-*

*wire. Many chronic diseases of lifestyle are the result of*

*imbalances in this node: high blood pressure, high cho-*

*lesterol, heart disease, type 2 diabetes, and anemia, to*

*name a few. Many women actively seek alternatives to*

*medication for treatment of imbalances in this node.*

*There are many options. The "right" choice is the one*

*that is realistic and effective for you and often changes*

*as your situation and stage in life change.*

THE CARDIOVASCULAR and lymphatic systems intimidate me. They are intricate, complex systems that people spend lifetimes studying. Despite my cursory understanding of them, I have found they are also fabulously receptive to lifestyle modifications. There is no other node in which lifestyle modifications stand to have the most impact.

"Chronic diseases of lifestyle" refers to long-term diseases that result because of lifestyle choices. These include:

- high blood pressure
- high cholesterol
- type 2 diabetes
- heart disease

Too many women chalk up their "disease" to family history, missing the opportunity to refine their lifestyle to have the health they want. For many, taking a pill is easier than changing their lifestyle.

Medication is the go-to medical treatment for chronic diseases of lifestyle. In the clinic, I see the women who don't want medication for high blood pressure, statin medication for high cholesterol, or metformin for type 2 diabetes. They seek me out for just this reason—solutions other than medication. Although there are nutrients and herbs that can be subbed out for medication—and nutrients, herbs, and medication all have their time and place—pill popping is not the entirety of our conversation. The bigger, more important conversation is about lifestyle.

Are you living the best you can? Are there things you could subtract, such as stress, hours in front of the television, and processed food? What about things you could add, such as movement, vegetables, and a daily practice, like meditation or yoga, that will support the life and health you want? How much responsibility are you willing to take for your choices?

The lymphatic system does the tremendous job of filtering our blood. Lymphatic drainage, a technique using light massage, helps promote the movement of lymphatic fluid to an area with working lymph vessels. It is commonly used to treat lymphedema, or swelling, in an arm after a woman has a mastectomy. An increasing number of massage therapists recognize the importance of lymph drainage, offering it as a treatment and teaching people the skill. We change the air filter, engine filter, and fuel filters in our cars. It makes perfect sense to me that we want and need to tend to our body's filter, our lymph, as well.

Sugar and insulin are transported around our bodies and, as such, influence so many aspects of our health. High blood sugar levels and high insulin levels cause inflammation, which is the root cause of many health issues. If I could teach one thing to the world, men and women, young and old, it would be the imperativeness of having stable blood sugar and insulin levels for good health. It is physiologically impossible to have high blood sugar and insulin levels and be healthy.

Heart disease is the primary cause of death for women, with higher rates for Black women than for white largely because of systemic racism and elevated stress levels. Thus, health in the Transport Node means reducing the largest cause of death. Functionally, you stand to enjoy an able body and your best life, free from disease. This is the value in balancing the Transport Node.

## Chronic Diseases of Lifestyle
. . . . . . . . . . . . . . . . . . . . . . . . . . . . .

### High blood pressure
At the clinic, when I take a woman's blood pressure and it is elevated, I ask her to take her blood pressure at home, first thing in the morning, for two weeks, and send me the results.

Stable blood
sugar and insulin levels
are **essential to
having good health.**

———————————

One elevated blood pressure reading is not necessarily indicative of a disease process. Dr. Mark Houston, a functional cardiologist from Nashville, considers an elevated nighttime blood pressure to be the most accurate indicator of risk of a cardiovascular event. Twenty-four-hour blood pressure testing is the most accurate way to diagnose hypertension as well as to determine the best course of treatment. I've never seen a patient diagnosed with high blood pressure who has been this thoroughly evaluated.

Elevated blood pressure is not a disease. When blood pressure is high, it means there are functional and structural abnormalities in the arterial system. To get to the root cause of high blood pressure, we must figure out *why* there are abnormalities in the arterial system. Receptors in the arterial wall ask the body whether what is entering the system is friend or foe. Abnormalities in the vascular system are generally responses to inflammation, oxidative stress, or autoimmune dysfunction. These responses are the result of something entering the system that should not be there, such as chemicals, toxins, pesticides, lipids, or sugar.

### Cholesterol

Cholesterol gets a bad rap, but it is a necessary molecule not only for hormone production but also for our cell membranes. Cholesterol gets into the body in two ways: it is either produced by the liver (75 percent) or absorbed from food (25 percent).

Not all "bad" cholesterol (known as LDL) is bad, and not all "good" cholesterol (known has HDL) is good. There are different kinds of LDL, some of which are not bad, and too high HDL is inflammatory. When there is high cholesterol, the question to ask is whether the cholesterol that is high is dangerous. If the cholesterol that is elevated is dangerous, the risk of forming blockages that can lead to a heart attack or stroke is increased.

## Heart disease

About one in sixteen women in the US have heart disease. For most people, it is preventable and reversible. Knowing your risk of heart disease, heart attack, stroke, diabetes, kidney disease, and inflammation is key to understanding your heart health. Heart disease is multifactorial: the combined risk factors of inflammation, metabolics (blood sugar and insulin in the blood), and genes determine whether or not people develop heart disease.

The artery wall lining can become inflamed for different reasons, such as poor diet or smoking. Inflammation weakens and scars the artery wall lining, making it easier for cholesterol to attach and form blockages called plaques. Inflammation also increases the risk of plaques breaking off and causing a clot, resulting in a heart attack or stroke.

When there is a lot of sugar in the blood, it damages the arterial walls, making it easier for cholesterol to get trapped and form a blockage. Blockages are not only the result of what we eat but also of our exposure to toxins and the health of our gut.

Our genes influence which medications, exercise, and nutrition can mitigate heart disease.

## Type 2 diabetes

Type 2 diabetes used to be known as adult-onset diabetes. The increase in childhood obesity, frequently the net result of the SAD and a sedentary lifestyle, has led to an increase in the incidence of type 2 diabetes in children.

Type 2 diabetes results when there is too much sugar circulating in the bloodstream. The pancreas does not produce enough insulin and cells respond poorly to insulin. Ultimately, cells take in less sugar. This leads to disorders of the circulatory, nervous, and immune systems.

## Insulin resistance

Insulin resistance occurs when insulin released from the pancreas does not work the way it's supposed to because the organs are blocking it from entering cells, thereby reducing its effects inside the cells. Insulin resistance is also sometimes called insulin block.

## Anemia

Anemia is a broad term that describes when there are not enough healthy red blood cells to carry oxygen to the body's tissues. When your tissues aren't absorbing enough oxygen, you feel tired and weak.

There are many forms of anemia, including, but not limited to, iron-deficiency anemia, vitamin deficiency anemia, and aplastic anemia. Different anemias have different causes, such as B12 deficiency, folate deficiency, certain medications, autoimmune disease, and nutrient malabsorption because of underlying gut issues. Determining the root cause of an anemia ensures effective treatment.

## She Was Game

Jenny is the poster child for functional medicine. This spritely seventy-nine-year-old married woman healed from candida and reversed her diagnosis of metabolic syndrome—the cluster of hypertension, hyperglycemia, excess body fat around the waist, and elevated cholesterol or triglyceride levels—over the course of only six months. She was willing to do whatever it took—overhaul her nutrition, exercise, take supplements, and revamp her wardrobe when nothing fit after significant weight loss. She was upbeat and positive. She happily shared her progress with her primary care doctor, who championed her effort and our work together.

Jenny was petite and 150 pounds when we met. She was referred to me by her primary care doctor to help her with chronic diarrhea. As is so often the case, because symptoms do not generally occur one at a time, because everything is connected to everything, Jenny came with a litany of other diagnoses, including type 2 diabetes, high blood pressure, high cholesterol, hypothyroidism, esophagitis, heartburn, and thrush. She did not want to take metformin, a medication prescribed to treat type 2 diabetes. She said what so many women do: "There must be something I can do. There must be another way, other than just taking medication." Indeed, there is.

When I asked Jenny what she had eaten in the last twenty-four hours, she reported consuming two slices of bread, mustard, four ounces of deli ham, raspberries, and diet orange soda; two soft boiled eggs, bread with butter, herbal tea, coffee with Coffee-Mate, and orange juice; rotisserie chicken and green beans, a bowl of fruit, and another diet orange soda. She routinely drank two diet sodas a day. She said this diet was a significant improvement from what she had been eating up until three days before. Prior to her recent effort, she typically had waffles for breakfast, candy after dinner, and cookies every day. She ate bread with dinner and canned fruit at lunch. By my estimation, her carbohydrate and sugar consumption were elevated, even with her recent modifications.

I was concerned that Jenny's health was threatened, that she was actively at risk of having a heart attack and stroke. I ordered a vitamin D3 test, a comprehensive metabolic panel (CMP) to evaluate her kidney and liver function, a food sensitivity panel to identify which foods were inflammatory for her, triggering or exacerbating the diarrhea, and a stool test to evaluate the health of her microbiome. I advised her to stop drinking diet soda, to stop using Coffee-Mate, and to eliminate bread completely. I was thinking that eliminating artificial sweeteners and non-food foods and significantly decreasing her daily carbohydrate consumption might yield significant improvements in a relatively short period of time. She was game.

## TRANSPORT NODE: CONVENTIONAL LABS

**Fasting and two-hour insulin and glucose.** A blood test measuring insulin and glucose levels first thing in the morning before eating and again after consuming a large amount of carbohydrates. Consuming a large amount of carbohydrates challenges the pancreas to make enough insulin to metabolize the carbohydrates. This blood test is the gold standard used to diagnose insulin resistance and type 2 diabetes.

**HgA1c.** A blood test that reflects blood sugar stability over the past three months.

**High-sensitivity C-reactive protein (hs-CRP).** A blood test for markers of systemic inflammation. Hs-CRP is a surrogate marker for interleukins, proteins made by white blood cells that regulate immune responses. Hs-CRP screens for infections and inflammatory diseases. It does not diagnose a specific disease.

**Homocysteine.** A blood test that measures this amino acid in the blood. Vitamins B6, B12, and folate are necessary to metabolize homocysteine, such that increased levels of the amino acid may be a sign of deficiency in those vitamins. High levels of homocysteine can damage the lining of the arteries and make the blood clot easily, increasing the risk of blood vessel blockages.

### TRANSPORT NODE: FUNCTIONAL LABS

**Advanced lipid testing.** A blood test that evaluates more specific lipoproteins than a standard cholesterol test to better assess cardiovascular disease risk. Testing includes measuring levels of different LDLs and HDLs, markers related to genetic risk of high cholesterol, and markers of inflammation.

**Cardiovascular genomics.** A blood draw or cheek swab that detects genetic polymorphisms associated with heart disease, high blood pressure, diabetes, atrial fibrillation, stroke, and high cholesterol.

**Comprehensive Nutritional Evaluation.** A blood and urine test used to evaluate the functional need for antioxidants, B vitamins, minerals, essential fatty acids, amino acids, digestive support, and other select nutrients. The test also screens for heavy metal toxicity. Micronutrient sufficiency is essential for optimal transport of nutrients and fluids throughout the body.

## Connecting Histories

Jenny grew up and had raised her own family in New England. She had worked part-time at a school and as a store clerk.

Jenny had an extensive surgical history. Multiple surgeries suggest significant antibiotic exposure. Antibiotics are routinely given during surgery to prevent infection. She'd had a kidney stone removed, a tubal ligation, a total hysterectomy, three cervical and two lumbar discectomies, an appendectomy, and rotator cuff repairs on both shoulders. She'd had breast cancer, and rectal bleeding from taking antibiotics. She was taking medications for heartburn, high blood pressure, and allergies.

Her family history was peppered with Transport Node issues: Her dad had heart disease and died from a heart attack when he was fifty-two years old. Her mom fell, had a stroke, and died at seventy-one years old. Her siblings died from complications due to Down syndrome, type 1 diabetes, pancreatic cancer, and morbid obesity. Autoimmune disease had a strong showing in Jenny's family, as well, by way of cancer and type 1 diabetes (more about autoimmune disease in chapter 10, on the Defense and Repair Node). Jenny's personal health history, nutrition history, surgical history, and family history all revealed significant contributing factors affecting her current health.

While undergoing treatment for candida, she had a car accident that necessitated rotator cuff surgery, during which time she was given two doses of insulin. Her primary care physician started her on "diabetes medication." She took one dose of metformin, which gave her watery diarrhea. She then threw away all the sugar in her house. She lost twelve pounds over four months simply by removing sugar from her diet.

Before her accident, Jenny walked regularly at the YMCA and did a lot of house and yard work. Her recent rotator cuff surgery limited her physical activity, as did the fatigue. She would do a few chores and then had to sit down to rest.

## TRANSPORT NODE: LIFESTYLE MODIFICATIONS

**Improve heart rate variability using HeartMath.** HeartMath sells tools designed to help people increase their heart rate variability. Increasing heart rate variability decreases the risk of heart disease and cardiovascular events, as well as yielding measurable benefits to our own and others' well-being.

**Exercise.** I recommend thirty minutes of aerobic exercise five days a week, plus two strength-training sessions per week. High-intensity interval training (HIIT) is ideal. Exercise increases BDNF, increases oxygenation, improves sleep, reduces stress, reduces fat, improves insulin sensitivity, and increases neuroplasticity. It raises serotonin, promotes sweating and detoxification, improves muscle mass, and promotes intestinal motility.

**Meditate.** Neurophysiological and neuroanatomical studies show that meditation can have long-standing effects on the brain, reducing the risk of cardiovascular disease. Meditation also reduces blood pressure.

**Avoid sugar, artificial sweeteners, and refined grains.** These foods have high glycemic impact, meaning they lead to sharp increases in blood sugar. High blood sugar contributes to inflammation, arterial disease, and insulin resistance.

**Eat lean protein and plant-based fat with every meal.** The glycemic impact of a food is how much that food boosts blood sugar. The total amount of carbohydrates consumed at a meal or snack largely determines what the blood sugar does. Coupling moderate glycemic foods with protein or fat reduces the glycemic impact of food, thereby reducing the glycemic impact of a meal.

**Do lymphatic drainage.** A manual technique that typically involves small circular motions designed to stimulate the flow of lymph, a fluid that transports white blood cells, oxygen, and nutrients throughout the body. This technique is usually offered by massage therapists, although you can learn to do it yourself too.

**How we live and what we eat** influence the expressions of our genes.

## Participation is Required to Reverse Disease

Two weeks after her first visit with me, Jenny returned, excited to review her test results. In the interim, she had a visit with her primary care physician. She told him she stopped metformin and planned to address her health through nutrition and exercise. To his credit, he supported her effort. Her stools normalized when she stopped taking metformin.

I wrote Jenny an exercise prescription, knowing she liked to walk. I encouraged her to start with walking for ten minutes, three times per week. Exercise was critical, I explained, as a lifestyle intervention to help stabilize her blood sugar and reduce her insulin. She started vitamin D3 supplementation based on her test results.

When she returned to the clinic three weeks later, she walked in and said, "I feel so much better." She had eliminated diet soda, was taking vitamin D3, and was walking a half mile six days a week. She said her next goal was to drink more water because she noticed her urine was "still yellow." I had taught her that the more yellow her urine, the more likely she was dehydrated and the more stress there was on her kidneys, which were already stressed because of her health issues.

It is simpler to think about what we *can* eat as opposed to what we *cannot* eat. Focusing on what we can't eat can be overwhelming and can feel oppressive for some. Gluten and dairy are the most common dietary culprits of functional bowel disease and inflammation. I advised Jenny to eat lean meat, vegetables except for nightshades (tomatoes, potatoes, peppers, and eggplant), fruit (mostly berries), coconut, and sweet potatoes for six weeks. Then, she could add nuts, seeds, and beans for another six weeks. This is a modified Autoimmune Protocol.

Jenny had labs done with her primary care physician, who appreciated her across-the-board improvement. He recommended repeating labs in three months. Unsurprisingly, her functional stool test showed yeast and bacterial overgrowth, for which I treated her. The test also showed she was deficient in bile acid, so I started her on bile salts and, for the digestive tract, an anti-inflammatory composed primarily of turmeric, rosemary leaf extract, and amino acids. I started her on a probiotic used specifically to treat yeast overgrowth.

At her next visit, Jenny said, "I'm fantastic. I have lots of energy. I feel absolutely normal. My bowel movements—I should take a picture. I go once a day. It's perfectly formed." In the last twenty-four-hours she'd had a five-grain flax wrap with turkey and lettuce, and water; plain almond milk yogurt, half a cup of frozen blueberries, half a cup of All-Bran Buds, half a grapefruit, and tea; chicken, asparagus, broccoli, and strawberries. She was sleeping well. She was going to the YMCA every day and walking the circumference of the track five times, which took her about sixteen minutes. She felt she could do more. Her blood pressure was normal. Her weight decreased from 150 pounds to 125. She went shopping and bought all new clothes. Her fasting blood sugar was still 120. We were aiming for ideal, which is less than 100. I encouraged her to stop eating fruit at night.

One month later, her vitamin D3 was normal and her average blood glucose decreased to 100. She was now walking a mile a day.

When I last saw Jenny, she had traveled to the West Coast to visit her extended family. She was joyful as she shared stories of time with her children and grandchildren. She talked about how hard it was to eat well when dining out. She was due for a physical exam with her primary care physician at the end of the summer and planned to repeat her labs. Her bowel movements were normal. Her energy was great. She was off all her medication. Her blood sugar was lower each time she had it tested.

Jenny did her part to reverse metabolic syndrome and type 2 diabetes without medication. Her added bonus was resolving her diarrhea. The long-term plan of care was for her to finish her therapeutic supplements, continue basic supplements, and maintain the lifestyle modifications she had put in place. Jenny worked every node of the matrix and reaped the benefits of her efforts.

## TRANSPORT NODE: NUTRITION INTERVENTIONS

**Follow the Cardiometabolic Diet.** The Cardiometabolic Diet is a modified Mediterranean diet developed by IFM, which recommends consuming whole, fresh, unprocessed foods such as fruits, vegetables, whole grains, nuts, legumes, dairy, extra-virgin olive oil, spices, and modest amounts of poultry, fish, red meat, and even red wine. The Cardiometabolic Diet has a low glycemic impact, targets calories that balance blood sugar, is high in fiber and low in simple sugars, incorporates balanced quality fats, and is rich in condition-specific phytonutrients.

**Eat fish.** Cold-water fish are rich in omega-3 fatty acids. Sardines, mackerel, anchovies, herring, and salmon are among the richest in the omega-3s. Large, oily fish like swordfish, tuna, and halibut have higher levels of mercury and are best eaten sparingly.

**Eat seeds.** Seeds like flax, chia, and hemp are rich, plant-based sources of omega-3 fatty acids. They are also high in protein and fiber. Include them all on a rotating basis.

**Eat walnuts.** Walnuts block intestinal absorption of cholesterol, are rich in antioxidants, and are high in fiber, protein, and omega-3 fatty acids.

**Season with cinnamon.** This spice is rich in cinnamaldehyde, a compound that helps regulate blood sugar.

**Add bonito flakes.** Bonito peptides have been shown to impact the formation of angiotensin II through their interaction with angiotensin-converting enzyme, supporting normal blood pressure.

## Supplements

**Bergamot.** Bergamot has been found to reduce cholesterol, triglycerides, and LDL. It has also been shown to increase HDL.

**CoQ10.** A potent antioxidant that protects and supports mitochondria. CoQ10 plays a central role in the electron transport chain of ATP production. CoQ10 supports cardiovascular health by inhibiting low-density lipoprotein oxidation, a chemical process that makes LDL inflammatory.

**Hawthorn.** A common shrub in the rose family. Hawthorn can improve the amount of blood pumped out of the heart, widen blood vessels, and increase the transmission of nerve signals. It is shown to lower blood pressure because it relaxes blood vessels. Hawthorn can lower cholesterol, LDL, and triglycerides. Hawthorn fruit extract may lower cholesterol by increasing the excretion of bile, reducing the formation of cholesterol, and enhancing the receptors for LDL.

**Omega-3 fatty acids.** Essential fats the body can't make but must get from food or supplementation. They are part of the cell membrane and affect the function of the receptors in cell membranes. They modulate contraction, relaxation, inflammation, and gene function.

**Red yeast rice.** The product of Monascus purpureus yeast grown on white rice. Red yeast rice contains compounds that appear to lower cholesterol levels. One of the compounds is monacolin K, the same ingredient that is in the cholesterol-lowering prescription drug lovastatin. Monacolin K can lower total blood cholesterol levels, LDL, and triglyceride levels.

## Your Genes Are Not Your Destiny

Women often attribute imbalances of the Transport Node to their family history. However, our genes are not our destiny. Just because we have a family history of high cholesterol doesn't mean we are destined to develop high cholesterol. How we live and what we eat influence the expressions of our genes. When lifestyle and nutritional modifications do not improve symptoms, supplements can further mitigate genetic influence on chronic diseases of lifestyle. There are a lot of tools in the toolbox.

# 10

# Immunity, Inflammation, and Infection

. . . . . . . . . . . . . . . . . .

### DEFENSE AND REPAIR NODE:
IMMUNE, INFLAMMATION,
INFECTION AND MICROBIOTA

AUTOIMMUNE DISEASE RESIDES *in the Defense and Repair Node, the intersection of gut health and immunity. Colitis, diverticulitis, tendonitis, vaginitis, sinusitis, cystitis, thyroiditis—the suffix "-itis" indicates inflammation is afoot. Resolving the root cause of inflammation resolves autoimmune disease and a host of other diseases. It's no longer enough to have a strong immune system. You need to cultivate immune resilience, which is, in essence, your ability to rebound from an insult to your immune system. How do you recover? As an increasing number of new viruses, toxins, and bacteria present, a balanced Defense and Repair Node is essential.*

COVID-19 MADE words like "cytokine storm," "interleukin," and "TH cell" part of everyday conversation. Once the proprietary language of immunologists, these elements of the Defense and Repair Node are now part of many people's everyday vernacular. COVID-19 illuminated how important having a healthy immune system is to our survival. The virus also shed light on the aspects of twenty-first century living that compromise a person's immune system and threaten their longevity. As a society, we are finally recognizing the value of nurses' work and childcare providers' services, but also of living at a slower pace, educating children outdoors, spending time in nature, having meaningful relationships, managing stress in healthy ways, eating unprocessed food, maintaining our mental health... Reprioritizing our values has come at a steep price for many but was sorely needed.

Treating the immune system is particularly challenging because of its complexity. But taking care of women and *not* tending to autoimmune disease is difficult, if not impossible, because of its prevalence. Autoimmune disease affects two women for every one man, and 25 percent of people with one autoimmune disease will develop another. I take care of the whole woman, which means I am taking care of her immune system as well.

During IFM's foundation course Applying Functional Medicine in Clinical Practice (AFMCP), I was introduced to the idea that 60 percent of the immune system resides in the gut, rendering gut health essential to immune system health. Whereas the Assimilation Node focuses on the degradation of barriers within the digestive system and the subsequent inflammation, the Defense and Repair Node homes in on the processes that occur *after* intestinal inflammation—the subsequent immune dysregulation and self-amplifying loop of systemic inflammation. I attended AFMCP in 2007. Years later, I met with a long-time functional chiropractic neurologist who drew me a picture of how the immune system works. He was a gracious teacher, but I left thinking, How am I ever going to remember all of that? Years later, I was reintroduced to T-cells—infection- and cancer-fighting cells—and I (finally) began to understand the basic workings of the immune system.

My knowledge of the immune system remains cursory. I am surprised time and time again by how applying principles of functional medicine—such as "start with the gut"—when caring for people with dysregulated immune systems so frequently yields significant improvement. Not 100 percent improvement, and certainly not 100 percent of the time, but often. Often enough to keep me going to work. The connection between our lifestyle and its effect on our immune system has been poorly understood and remains poorly understood by many, particularly those practicing conventional medicine. It seems that the primary interventions conventional medical practitioners have to offer people with compromised immune systems are steroids and immunosuppressant medications. These medications save lives, yet they frequently stop working, and the "why" of a dysregulated immune system is rarely addressed.

That people with "compromised immune systems" and "comorbidities" were at greater risk of getting COVID and got sicker from it seems to have awakened the medical community and society to the relationship between immune system health with the incidence and severity of disease. Collectively, we are now more invested in understanding the variables that influence sickness and disease. COVID has shown us hyper-hygiene is not the answer.

Many people are sick with unnamable illnesses—constellations of symptoms that don't fit tidily into established medical diagnoses. Women to Women was a beacon for those people. Women would come from all over the world, having been to

Immune system disease can **go into remission.**

---

world-renowned medical institutions like the Mayo Clinic, Johns Hopkins, and Dana-Farber, having had executive work-ups but feeling no better for their evaluations and treatments. The more I learn about the immune system, the more riveted I am by it. I suspect I will spend the rest of my life learning what I can, digesting the information, and then going back for more. It is layered and complicated: the intersection of gut health, inflammation, micronutrient sufficiency, genetics, detoxification, and a cascade of biochemical reactions that can be interrupted at numerous junctions but *must* be interrupted if wellness is going to be recovered. Which it can be. And perhaps this is the most profound thing I've learned about the immune system: immune system disease can go into remission. You can avoid certain substances, you can eat certain foods, you can take supplements and plant medicines that can help. This diverges from conventional medical messaging that if you are sick because of your immune system, you are sick for life. That immune system disease can go into remission offers people *hope*, perhaps the most powerful medicine of all.

The conversation around immune system health has evolved into a discussion about immune system resilience—the capacity to adapt to challenges by establishing, maintaining, and regulating an appropriate immune response. Immune system resilience requires flexibility and adaptability.

I've contemplated resilience for a long time: What is the difference between sexually active young women who use contraception and those who do not? Why are some sexual-trauma survivors disabled by their experience while for others the trauma fuels their work, art, poetry, or life? Why do some people lose a ski race and throw a ski pole in the snow while others figure out how they can ski faster next time? Why are some women who lose a child unable to get out of bed while others can keep going? Why do some people who lose a parent when they are a child go on to live a healthy lifestyle while others become addicts? What are the characteristics we can nurture in ourselves and each other that lead to emotional *and* physical flexibility and adaptability, so we can navigate life's challenges in as healthy a way as possible and live as well as we can?

Other emerging concepts in the field of immunology include immunorejuvenation. Our immune system sounds an alarm when we are exposed to things like toxins or viral infection. The memory of that exposure gets encoded in the genetic programming of our immune system, controlling how the immune system functions. This gets communicated from cell to cell, manifesting as too much response—in other words, inflammation—or too little response—immune suppression. A balanced immune system can adapt to the situation at hand. The body rejuvenates its immune system through a process called autophagy. Autophagy removes damaged cells coded with the memory of exposure, allowing cells without a built-in alarm to take over, leading to a balanced or rejuvenated immune system.

Immunosenescence refers to the changes to the immune system associated with aging. Factors such as genetics, nutrition, exercise, previous exposure to microorganisms, and biological and cultural sex influence immunosenescence. While we can't stop aging, we can influence some of its effect on our immune system through lifestyle choices.

*Life* is possible with relative health in the Defense and Repair Node. Living with the vulnerability of a compromised immune system is terrifying. The whole world can feel unsafe if you never know what straw will break the camel's back and trigger a flare. To live life without fear—of viruses, bacteria, foods, people, places, and toxins—is freedom, a freedom easily taken for granted by those of us who are well, whose immune systems are flexible and able to adapt to what the world throws our way.

## "Itis" Means Inflammation

A diagnosis ending in "-itis" is indicative of an imbalance in the Defense and Repair Node. "Itis" is a suffix that means inflammation:

* colitis
* diverticulitis
* tendonitis
* vaginitis
* sinusitis
* bursitis
* dermatitis
* thyroiditis

The home of inflammation is in the gut, and unstopped inflammation activates the immune system. If the inflammation and activation of the immune system are unstopped, the cycle continues indefinitely.

Triggers causing intestinal inflammation include toxins, proteins, pathogens, lipopolysaccharides (bacterial toxins), alcohol, and stress. Intestinal inflammation can damage the mucosa lining the intestines, compromise the intestinal barrier, resulting in leaky gut, or activate the immune system. In leaky gut, the impermeable membrane lining the intestines becomes permeable.

Some immune reactions are associated with chronic inflammatory disease, including:

* allergies
* asthma
* reduced oral tolerance such as food allergies or celiac disease
* autoimmune disease

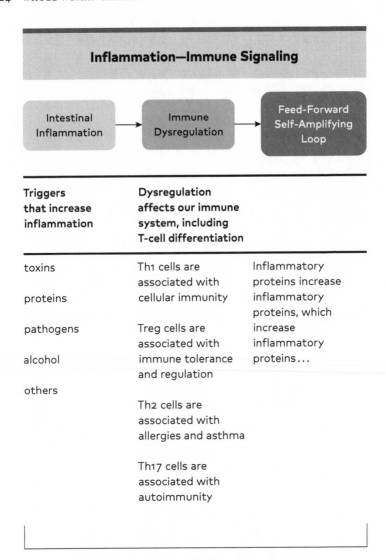

## Inflammation—Immune Signaling

| Intestinal Inflammation | Immune Dysregulation | Feed-Forward Self-Amplifying Loop |
| --- | --- | --- |

| Triggers that increase inflammation | Dysregulation affects our immune system, including T-cell differentiation | |
| --- | --- | --- |
| toxins | Th1 cells are associated with cellular immunity | Inflammatory proteins increase inflammatory proteins, which increase inflammatory proteins... |
| proteins | | |
| pathogens | Treg cells are associated with immune tolerance and regulation | |
| alcohol | | |
| others | | |
| | Th2 cells are associated with allergies and asthma | |
| | Th17 cells are associated with autoimmunity | |

**These three pathways lead to tissue damage**

Some people do not get better even after an inflammatory trigger is removed. We have to reduce a protein complex called NF-kB, which copies DNA to express inflammation, so that there is less DNA damage and less production of inflammatory proteins. Tissue damage occurs systemically until the cycle of NF-kB production is stopped. The feed forward, self-amplifying loop of NF-kB is the mechanism by which people stay stuck in disease and develop multiple autoimmune diseases.

## Uncovering Triggers, Uncovering Layers

Five years post-menopause and fifty-five years old, Petra had four autoimmune disease diagnoses and a team of specialists working with her when we met. Her team included an acupuncturist, a cranial sacral therapist, a rheumatologist, a cardiologist, a gastroenterologist, a pulmonologist, and a primary care physician. She sought my help because, despite her team and extensive medical workups, she was "still having issues."

It all started with the relatively uneventful birth of her second son. Petra developed a rash and nothing was the same since. She developed migraines with aura, constipation, asthma, and fatigue. She developed numbness in her face and left arm and was ultimately diagnosed with celiac disease. Next came her diagnosis of mixed connective tissue disease, then skin lupus, and then autoimmune thyroiditis.

Her symptoms included joint pain, muscle pain, itching, rashes, nasal congestion, fatigue, constipation, and depression. Petra was also experiencing night sweats, a decreased sex drive, and vaginal dryness. Her goals were specific: to be able to travel internationally to visit her son, to decrease her respiratory symptoms, to increase her energy, to decrease her hormone symptoms, and to stop or slow the autoimmune cascade running rampant throughout her body.

We looked at her health history using the Functional Medicine Timeline and went all the way back to her infancy. We noted that Petra was bottle fed as an infant; she missed out on the benefits of immune globulin–rich breast milk, which inoculates our intestines with beneficial bacteria and sets the stage for our immune systems to properly function. She had recurrent ear infections and strep throat as a child, suggesting an undiagnosed dairy sensitivity, and recurrent antibiotic exposure. She'd had mononucleosis in the past. Her dad was in the military, so she lived in many different countries growing up. Living around the world increased her exposure to bacteria and viruses. All of these factors set her up for a dysregulated immune system.

Petra's family health history suggested a genetic predisposition for autoimmune disease, as well: her mom had hypothyroidism, her dad had hypercholesterolemia and progressive myelopathy, and her maternal grandmother had cancer.

Our work together included food sensitivity testing, a stool test, and a Comprehensive Nutritional Evaluation. Her stool test results showed her immune system was compromised, she was not optimally digesting fat, and she had dysbiosis and yeast. Her food sensitivity testing showed prolific sensitivities and allergies to eggs, milk, peanuts, sesame, and tomatoes. She started digestive enzymes, a multivitamin, high-dose glutamine, botanical yeast treatment, and high-dose fish oil. She eliminated foods that tested inflammatory and allergenic for her.

## DEFENSE AND REPAIR NODE:
## CONVENTIONAL LABS

**Thyroglobulin antibody (TgAb).** A blood test that measures antibodies to a protein called thyroglobulin. This protein is found in thyroid cells. Thyroglobulin antibodies can be a sign of thyroid gland damage caused by the immune system.

**CD57.** A blood test measuring the CD57 marker, which is present on natural killer cells and T cells. In cases of chronic disease, including Lyme, the number of CD57 cells has been shown to be low. The utility of this test is controversial.

**Complete blood count with differential (CBC with differential).** A blood test used to evaluate overall health and detect a wide range of disorders. The differential evaluates white blood cells, which are elements of the immune system. This can help identify what is taxing the immune system. For example, eosinophil cells become active in the later stages of inflammation. These white blood cells respond to allergic and parasitic disease. One-third of the body's histamine is found in the eosinophilic cell.

**High-sensitivity C-reactive protein (hs-CRP).** A blood test for markers of systemic inflammation. Hs-CRP is a surrogate marker for interleukins, proteins made by white blood cells that regulate immune responses. Hs-CRP screens for infections and inflammatory diseases. It does not diagnose a specific disease.

**Interleukin 6 (IL-6).** A blood test for IL-6, a protein made by various cells. IL-6 helps regulate immune responses and thus is a marker of immune system activation. It can be elevated with inflammation, infection, autoimmune disorders, heart disease, and some cancers.

**Thyroid peroxidase antibody (TPOAb).** A blood test that measures thyroid peroxidase normally found in the thyroid gland. TPO plays an important role in the production of thyroid hormones. TPOAb detects antibodies against TPO in the blood, suggesting that the cause of thyroid disease is an autoimmune disorder like autoimmune thyroiditis or Graves' disease.

### DEFENSE AND REPAIR NODE: FUNCTIONAL LABS

**Intestinal permeability test.** A urinary test that measures the excretion of sugars and their ratio as a basis for measuring intestinal permeability.

**Pathogen-associated immune reactivity screen.** A blood test used to detect latent microorganisms that can cause disease, contributing to an immune system load.

**Stool testing.** A one-day stool collection, done at home, measuring gastrointestinal microbiota DNA. The test detects parasites, bacteria, fungi, and more. It measures indicators of digestion, absorption, inflammation, and immune function.

**Zonulin.** A protein that modulates the permeability of tight junctions between cells of the wall of the digestive tract. The junctions control the equilibrium between tolerance and immunity. Considered to be the biologic door to inflammation, autoimmunity, and cancer.

## Sometimes Things Get Worse before They Get Better

When it came to her health, Petra was varsity level: She had a lot of understanding about how food and lifestyle affected her health. She was already avoiding foods she knew made

"Itis" is a suffix that means **inflammation.**

her feel worse—dairy, alcohol, and grains. She was moving her body regularly through yoga and walking, she had a daily spiritual practice of meditation, her home and marriage were safe havens for her, she had good relationships with her sons and a network of friends for support, and she slept well. Her modifiable lifestyle factors were as good as they could be.

She had an appointment with her neurologist for ongoing numbness on the left side of her face. She had a brain MRI and an EMG, which were normal. She had blood work done, which showed elevated B6 and magnesium. She was advised by the neurologist to stop the multivitamin. He was concerned the elevated B6 was a cause of her numbness. She had been following our plan of care for three weeks and felt "drunk." She also was constipated. We discussed the possibility her symptoms might be a Herxheimer reaction, a short-term worsening of symptoms at the initiation of treatment, before improvement.

## DEFENSE AND REPAIR NODE: LIFESTYLE MODIFICATIONS

**Manage stress.** Chronic stress suppresses immune function. It decreases immune cell count and increases cytokine production. The physiologic effect of stress can be decreased through practices such as mindfulness, yoga, and monitoring heart rate variability.

**Meditate daily.** Daily meditation improves immune function.

**Exercise.** I recommend thirty minutes of aerobic exercise five days a week, plus two strength-training sessions per week. Exercise increases the immune system's T cells and natural killer cells. Exercise also lowers levels of inflammatory proteins called cytokines, which include interferons, interleukins, and growth factors.

**Sleep.** Sleeping seven to eight hours a night is ideal. Anti-inflammatory cytokines are made while we sleep, protecting us from inflammation and infection.

**Avoid harmful substances.** Avoid all tobacco products and limit alcohol intake.

**Handwash regularly.** This significantly decreases exposure to infectious pathogens.

## Evolving Processes

A few days later, Petra was feeling much better, though napping a lot. She said, "Neurology has no idea why I have neuropathy." Her energy was increasing and her brain was less foggy. She felt her improvement was most likely the result of eliminating inflammatory foods. She reflected on how she often ate the same foods day after day and needed to work on food rotation. She had not used her inhaler in months. She resumed magnesium because it helped with her constipation.

Ultimately, Petra opted not to travel internationally to see her son. She was reticent to do anything that might compromise her health. She worked hard for her improvement. She joined a gym and considered part-time employment. She hadn't worked in more than a year and a half. Eventually, she returned to work full-time and loved it.

## DEFENSE AND REPAIR NODE: NUTRITION INTERVENTIONS

**Eat the rainbow.** Eating foods of varying color every day supports all the nodes. Foods rich in color have high levels of antioxidants. The more colorful the foods you consume, the more antioxidants you get. Foods with different colors are phytonutrient rich in different ways. Phytonutrient diversity is key to optimal health. Eating the same foods every day limits nutrient availability. Ask yourself, have I eaten red foods today? orange? yellow? green? For blue foods, think blueberries, blue potatoes, and elderberries; for purple, think purple kale, eggplant, and purple cabbage.

**Eat fermented vegetables and other probiotic-containing foods.** Rich in pre- and probiotics, foods such as yogurt, kefir, sauerkraut, and kimchi help maintain gut barrier function essential for a balanced immune system.

**Eliminate (or reduce) sugar, processed carbohydrates, and excessive saturated fat.** These foods are immune-system offenders. Examples include sweet carbonated beverages, Goldfish crackers, butter, cheese, and fatty cuts of meat like bacon and salami.

**Use apple cider vinegar.** Apple cider vinegar is a natural antimicrobial. It inhibits the growth of bacteria high in lipopolysaccharides, toxins that cause leaky gut, a major contributor to immune system dysregulation.

**Consume bone broth.** Bone broth is rich in minerals, collagen, and amino acids. It supports connective tissue, joints, gut healing, muscle building, and mood. It is also rich in glucosamine, which helps repair leaky gut.

### Supplements

**Curcumin.** A potent antiviral and anti-inflammatory. Curcumin dampens NF-kB signaling.

**Epigallocatechin gallate (EGCG).** The phytonutrient found in green tea with strong antiviral and anti-inflammatory properties.

**Himalayan tartary buckwheat.** A plant grown in the Himalayan regions of China, India, and Nepal, and in a few places in the United States. Rich in 2-HOBA, also known as salicylamine, which has been shown to extend life and protect the body's proteins and fats against damage.

**Melatonin.** Primarily thought of to support sleep, melatonin has strong antiviral action and inhibits inflammation as well.

**N-acetylcysteine (NAC).** The supplement form of cysteine, which provides sulfur for glutathione production, replenishing glutathione stores. Glutathione supports normal immune function.

**Quercetin.** Proven to have strong antiviral effects against influenza, coronavirus, and herpesvirus, it also functions as an antioxidant and an anti-inflammatory, promoting healing.

**Resveratrol.** A potent antiviral and anti-inflammatory nutrient. The phytoalexin present in red wine, it provides cardioprotective, chemoprotective, and anti-inflammatory benefits. Resveratrol improves vascular function, extends the lifespan, has anti-aging effects, opposes the effects of high-calorie diets, mimics the effects of calorie restriction, and improves cellular function. Resveratrol provides protection against chemical, cholestatic, and alcohol injury to the liver. It decreases liver fibrosis and steatosis.

## When Your Life Depends on It

Despite health authorities waffling at the beginning of the COVID pandemic, mask-wearing became a key public health recommendation to stave off the spread of the disease. Mask-wearing quickly became a divisive, politicized topic. Over time, even those who once masked regularly changed their habits.

But some people mask out of necessity as opposed to choice: their life depends on it.

Having a healthy immune system—one that neither overreacts nor underreacts—allows you to move freely about the planet with a lot less fear than if your immune system is compromised. Immune resilience enables you to meet life's offenses and recover without life-altering impact to your health, whether you have encountered a virus, an insect sting, a bacterial infection, or a stressor. It's been said before, and it bears repeating: the way we interact with and live in our environment is a major determinant of our health, both as individuals and as a collective.

# 11

# Membranes, Bones, and Mechanics

. . . . . . . . . . . . . . . . . . .

*STRUCTURAL INTEGRITY NODE:*
*SUBCELLULAR MEMBRANES,*
*MUSCULOSKELETAL STRUCTURE*

SOMETIMES THE ROOT *cause of a health issue relates to the body's physical structure. Some issues within this node can be modified through lifestyle, some cannot. Sometimes arthritis is the result of an inflammatory process; sometimes it is the result of bone rubbing on bone. Some musculoskeletal pain is the result of an inflammatory process; sometimes it is anatomic, like scoliosis. The breadth of the Structural Integrity Node is vast, from skeleton to cell. The structural integrity of membranes includes the intestinal lining, the blood-brain barrier, and even cellular membranes. Each cell's membrane must be intact for optimal function.*

I TOOK care of a woman who suffered from severe constipation and did *everything*—for years—to try to resolve it. She tried multiple rounds of the Anti-Candida Food Plan, she took supplements out the wazoo, and she even avoided tomatoes—in August!—all to minimal avail. Eventually, she had a colonoscopy and was diagnosed with a "tortured colon," meaning her colon twisted. The anatomy of her colon was the variable contributing to her constipation we could not change. This explained why, despite her gallant efforts, her constipation largely persisted. Avoiding all the sugar in the world would not straighten her colon. She had a Structural Integrity Node issue.

Structure informs function. A basic tenet in biology and physiology, this summarizes that the way something is made affects the way it works. If something is made incorrectly, or not ideally, or the shape of it changes, function changes too.

One of the clinical skills taught in midwifery school is pelvimetry: the anatomy of a woman's pelvis is assessed to determine the ease (or lack thereof) with which a baby will be born. When the structure of the pelvis is "normal," it is deemed to be conducive to birth. If it is "abnormal," or there are prominent bones, a more difficult birth is anticipated. The anatomy of the pelvis is but one of many structural variables that affects the birthing process.

As my scope of practice has broadened over the years, I have had to expand my thinking about structure and function beyond the bony pelvis. The concerns women bring to the clinic necessitate I do so. No specialty captivates the relationship between structure and function as well as functional neurology.

## Functional Neurology
.........................

I've been interested in neurology ever since my father died from an inconveniently located brain tumor (not that brain tumors are ever conveniently located) at the age of sixty-six. His first brain surgery, at the age of fifty-one, was an attempt to remove as much of the tumor from his brain stem as possible. He had experienced profound weight gain, sleep apnea, and physical instability. He was unable to work for the first time in his life. After surgery, there was radiation followed by a whole litany of side effects. Recurrent aspiration pneumonia from his inability to swallow properly compromised his health. Whether his difficulty swallowing was the result of the tumor pressing on his brain stem or from radiation damage, we'll never know. He had a second surgery more than a decade later because the tumor had grown; he never recovered.

I don't believe functional neurology could have saved my father, but functional neurologists have an entirely different skill set from neurologists. Functional neurologists treat neurological disorders based on function. They use brain exercises and specific adjustments to improve the function of the nervous system that cannot be improved by surgery.

In a required course for my functional medicine certification, Dr. Datis Kharrazian taught how some physical symptoms can be traced to the function of specific parts of the brain. Exercises that work specific parts of the brain can ultimately restore function in other parts of the body. Eureka! Symptoms like difficulty swallowing, vertigo, imbalance, and ringing in the ears can all be improved by doing different types of exercises that strengthen the part of the brain that controls function. Functional neurology has a lot to offer for a variety of symptoms, whether it's post-concussion syndrome, vertigo, seizures, or small intestinal bacterial overgrowth (SIBO).

## The Web Is Complex
. . . . . . . . . . . . . . . . . . . . . .

Muscle pain (myalgia) and joint pain (arthralgia) are common symptoms women have when they come to the clinic. Sometimes they already have diagnoses of fibromyalgia, polymyalgia rheumatica, or rheumatoid arthritis. Sometimes they have chronic low back and neck pain. Our muscles and joints are vulnerable to pro-inflammatory cytokines. As you know from reading about the Defense and Repair Node, high levels of pro-inflammatory cytokines cause immune system imbalances. Sometimes inflammation and immune system activation manifest as musculoskeletal pain. Sometimes musculoskeletal pain is purely anatomic—bones rubbing on bones, ligaments torn or stretched, or skeletal misalignment.

The Structural Integrity Node encompasses the integrity of muscles and joints as well as membranes. Because of the involvement of membranes, structural imbalances go beyond the musculoskeletal system. All Structural Integrity imbalances overlap with other nodes in the matrix. For example, increases in intestinal permeability (leaky gut) are associated with eczema, inflammatory bowel disease, and several types of arthritis. The increase in intestinal permeability promotes the absorption of large nutrients from the intestines into the bloodstream, which can lead to the development of immune complexes, which leads to immune dysfunction, which can exacerbate musculoskeletal inflammation. In other words, a leaky gut leads to large nutrient absorption, leading to immune system activation, which triggers joint pain.

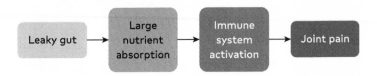

The web is complex: Excess estrogen, low testosterone, and low DHEA are common in women with rheumatic disorders. Correction of autoimmune thyroiditis may also alleviate inflammatory musculoskeletal disorders, including adhesive capsulitis. Brain inflammation is a major contributor to joint inflammation and cartilage degeneration. According to IFM literature, musculoskeletal pain and inflammation can cause three types of secondary depression:

- Inflammatory mediators released from degenerative tissues and system inflammation have psychoactive effects that contribute to fatigue, lethargy, anxiety, depression, dementia, and psychosis.

- Pain limits peoples' pursuits of pleasure.

- Decreased motility can result in isolation, increasing mental and emotional distress.

Inflammation is a common, albeit insidious, underwriter of structural imbalances. A functional medicine treatment approach to structural imbalances involves addressing the root cause of inflammation as opposed to simply suppressing the inflammation and pain. How is this done? By healing the gut.

## The Hip Bone's Connected to the . . .

Benita was a sixty-six-year-old retired health-care worker and mother of four. I met her in 2018 not long after she fell and broke her hip. She was concerned about her future health. She was experiencing joint pain, arthritis, vaginal dryness, painful sex, and fatigue. She was diagnosed with osteopenia in 2007 and took alendronic acid, also known as Fosamax, a conventional medical treatment for osteoporosis, for two years. Her most recent bone density test showed osteopenia in her spine.

Nothing protects
the health
of the bones like
**estrogen.**

---

She had open heart surgery for an atrial septal defect. She was taking a beta blocker to manage her atrial fibrillation. She had a history of endometriosis, ovarian cysts, gall bladder removal, and a fractured femur. Her dad died from colon cancer when she was twelve years old. Two of her children had lupus, two tested positive for antiphospholipid antibodies. All of which is to say, Benita's genetic potential for autoimmune disease and cancer was clear. Her family history also included high blood pressure, heart disease, stroke, and hyperparathyroidism.

The World Health Organization criteria for osteoporosis is based on women who are five-foot-five and weigh 150 pounds. This criteria is biased against petite women. A woman who is shorter and weighs less is essentially predisposed to having a diagnosis of osteoporosis. There is controversy around whether osteopenia should be a diagnosis at all.

Then there is the question of what to do about the test results. If someone is diagnosed with osteoporosis or has documented bone loss based on their own bone densities, I am not going to recommend bisphosphonate medication like Fosamax. In general, bisphosphonate medication is poorly tolerated by women. Some studies have shown it to *increase* the risk of fracture because it makes bone rigid and more likely to break, as opposed to bone's natural state, which has some flexibility. Bisphosphonate use is correlated with increased incidences of osteonecrosis of the jawbone and, in my clinical experience, the incidences are much greater than the studies show. A deteriorating jawbone makes it difficult to retain teeth, making it difficult to eat, compounding weight and muscle loss commonly experienced by women as we age.

Benita and I talked about doing a test to evaluate for active bone loss. We discussed testing her vitamin D3 levels, a vitamin necessary for bone formation, as well as running a Comprehensive Nutritional Evaluation to evaluate nutrient deficiencies, a hormone panel, and advanced lipid testing.

## STRUCTURAL INTEGRITY NODE:
## CONVENTIONAL LABS

**High-sensitivity C-reactive protein (hs-CRP).** A blood test for markers of systemic inflammation. Hs-CRP is a surrogate marker for interleukins, proteins made by white blood cells that regulate immune responses. Hs-CRP screens for infections and inflammatory diseases. It does not diagnose a specific disease.

**Pyridinium crosslinks.** A urine test done first thing in the morning to evaluate active bone loss. Can be used pre- and post-intervention to evaluate the effectiveness of a treatment.

**RA (rheumatoid arthritis) factor.** Tests for antibodies directed against rheumatoid factors (RFS), which are a marker for rheumatoid arthritis and other autoimmune conditions, although levels increase with age.

**Rheumatoid panel.** Typically includes hs-CRP, citrullinated peptide antibodies, IgA, and IgG. IgA and IgG are produced by the immune system and are directed against cyclic citrullinated peptides. Citrulline is naturally produced in the body as part of the metabolism of the amino acid arginine. In joints with rheumatoid arthritis, this conversion may happen at a higher rate.

**Sedimentation rate (sed rate or ESR).** A blood test that reveals inflammatory activity in the body.

**Vitamin D3.** A blood test measuring vitamin D3 levels in the body. Two forms of vitamin D are important for nutrition: D2 and D3. Vitamin D2 mainly comes from fortified foods like breakfast cereals, milk, and other dairy items. Vitamin D3 is made by your body when you are exposed to sunlight.

It is also found in some foods, including eggs and fatty fish, such as salmon, tuna, and mackerel. Vitamin D is essential for healthy bones and teeth.

## Imaging

**Bone density.** X-rays used to determine the nutrient density of bones, thereby determining the risk of breaking one. X-rays use radiation to create pictures of the inside of the body. Different tissue absorbs different amounts of radiation. Calcium in bones absorb X-rays the most, so bones look white. Air absorbs the least, so lungs look black.

**Computerized axial tomography (CAT scan).** Special X-rays that produce cross-sectional images of the body using X-rays and a computer.

**Magnetic resonance imaging (MRI).** An imaging technique that uses a magnetic field and radio waves to produce cross-sectional images that allow a view inside the body. Often used to evaluate soft tissues such as the brain, liver, and abdominal organs, as well as to visualize more subtle abnormalities not apparent on regular X-ray.

**Thermogram.** A test that uses an infrared camera to detect heat patterns and blood flow in body tissues.

## STRUCTURAL INTEGRITY NODE: FUNCTIONAL LABS

**2-, 4-, 16alpha-hydroxyestrone.** A urine test that measures the metabolites 2, 4, and 16alpha-hydroxyestrone. Estrogen is metabolized first in the gut and then in liver. In the liver, estrogen gets broken down into 2, 4, and 16alpha-hydroxyestrone: 2-hydroxyestrone protects against osteoporosis and nothing protects the health of the bones like estrogen. You can influence the way your body breaks down estrogen with things like exercise, flaxseed, and eating cruciferous vegetables.

**Comprehensive Nutritional Evaluation.** A blood and urine test used to evaluate the functional need for antioxidants, B vitamins, minerals, essential fatty acids, amino acids, digestive support, and other select nutrients. The test also screens for heavy metal toxicity and measures micronutrients essential for optimal ATP production.

**Intestinal permeability test.** A urinary test that measures the excretion of sugars and their ratio as a basis for measuring intestinal permeability. Osteoporosis is thought to have a gut-related component in that if we don't absorb the nutrients we need from our food, our body will take it from the nutrient reserve of our bones, contributing to bone loss.

**Stool testing.** A one-day stool collection, done at home, measuring gastrointestinal microbiota DNA. The test detects parasites, bacteria, fungi, and more. It measures indicators of digestion, absorption, inflammation, and immune function. A healthy gut ensures optimal nutrient absorption from our food, contributing to bone health.

## Structuring a Healthy Life

Benita exercised twenty minutes a day, six days per week. She enjoyed spending time outdoors, gardening, and sewing. Her twenty-four-hour diet recall included organic eggs and toast with fruit, one cup of coffee (which she drank daily); salad for lunch; and meat twice a week for dinner, some cheese, and some vegan entrées. She did not eat fast food and had little processed food. She snacked on candy and baked goods, which she craved, along with chocolate, which is largely thought to make the blood acidic, which contributes to bone loss.

An alkaline diet is central to treating osteoporosis. Daily urine pH strips can be used at home to assess whether or not this goal is being attained. Conventional recommendations for bone health include regular calcium supplementation and dairy consumption. I caution against this as too much calcium can contribute to kidney stone formation particularly in post-menopausal women. The best source of dietary calcium is leafy dark green vegetables. Vitamins D3 and K and the mineral strontium have been proved to generate new bone growth.

## STRUCTURAL INTEGRITY NODE: LIFESTYLE MODIFICATIONS

**Do high resistance exercise and other strength training.** Weight-bearing exercise has been shown to promote new bone growth, as well as decrease the incidences of high blood pressure, high cholesterol, heart disease, type 2 diabetes, and depression. High resistance exercise decreases inflammation and promotes lymphatic flow. It also increases muscle protein synthesis. Lift weights or do body weight exercise for at least thirty minutes twice a week.

**Receive regular massage.** Massage provides manual release of tension, decreases muscle contractions, stimulates lymph, and can promote relaxation and quieting of the central nervous system, thereby decreasing cortisol and subsequent pro-inflammatory cytokine production.

**Receive regular manipulation.** Chiropractic and osteopathic manipulation aligns organs as well as bones for optimal function.

**Practice daily meditation and relaxation.** Meditation and relaxation decrease cortisol. Decreasing cortisol essentially decreases inflammation. Less inflammation decreases the likelihood of joint pain.

**Try neuromuscular electrical stimulation.** A procedure in which small electric impulses are used to stimulate muscles that are weak or paralyzed. Neuromuscular electrical stimulation increases muscle strength, blood circulation, and range of motion. It also lessens muscle spasms. Also called NES, NMES, and therapeutic (subthreshold) electrical stimulation.

## Solidifying the Foundation, Protecting the Bones

When Benita and I spoke two months after her first visit, she had recently seen her cardiologist and had a chiropractor test her cortisol level. Initially she thought her cortisol level was low, but when we reviewed it, we determined it was normal. I encouraged her to add high-dose fish oil and chia, flax, and hemp seeds to her diet, and to increase her exercise.

A year and a half later, Benita came to the clinic for an annual exam. She was seeing her cardiologist routinely. She wanted to consider hormone therapy for many of her symptoms as well as for her bones. Nothing protects the health of the bones like estrogen. When the benefits of estrogen therapy outweigh the risks for an individual, estrogen is worth considering for the treatment of osteoporosis. Estrogen had potential benefits for treating Benita's hormonal symptoms and protecting her heart, in addition to her bone health.

Benita's osteoporosis is a classic example of how musculoskeletal issues overlap with other nodes in the matrix. Her gall bladder removal suggested Assimilation Node involvement;

When structural integrity is optimized, **optimal physical health is possible.**

———————————

her family history suggested Transport and Defense and Repair Node involvement; and her menopausal symptoms suggested Communication Node involvement.

I continue to work with her on solidifying her foundation—getting adequate exercise and eating optimally—to minimize her bone loss.

## STRUCTURAL INTEGRITY NODE: NUTRITION INTERVENTIONS

**Eat fish twice a week.** The bones of small fish such as anchovies and sardines are rich in protein, calcium, and omega-3 fatty acids, contributing to healthy bones.

**Eat lots of leafy dark green vegetables.** These are the best dietary source of calcium. They are also rich in vitamin K, which supports new bone growth.

**Eat grass-fed beef.** Grass-fed beef is rich in protein and vitamin B12.

**Consume bone broth.** Bone broth is rich in minerals, collagen, and amino acids. It supports connective tissue, joints, gut healing, muscle building, and mood.

**Eliminate alcohol, sugar, and processed foods.** These foods acidify the body and contribute to bone and ligament deterioration.

### Supplements

**Antioxidants.** Antioxidants like vitamin C and vitamin E decrease oxidative stress, improve mitochondrial function, and decrease the deterioration of cartilage.

**Bromelain.** An anti-inflammatory, helps decrease the pain of osteoarthritis.

**Calcium.** Builds bone, protects against excessive bone loss, helps blood to clot and muscles to contract, which includes helping our hearts to beat. Have serum levels tested prior to supplementation to be sure they are not high. A study of post-menopausal women taking routine calcium supplementation showed an increased incidence of kidney stones.

**Niacinamide.** A form of vitamin B3 used to treat osteoarthritis.

**Omega-3 fatty acids.** Essential fats the body can't make but must get from food or supplementation. They are part of the cell membrane and affect the function of the receptors in cell membranes. They modulate contraction, relaxation, inflammation, and gene function. They decrease joint pain and inflammation.

**Vitamin C.** Protects the breakdown of collagen, a process that can otherwise lead to joint swelling and pain.

**Vitamin D3.** Anti-inflammatory, pain reliever, and mood stabilizer that assists in calcium absorption and promotes new bone development.

**Vitamin K.** Has a positive effect on bone mineral density and reducing fracture risk. It comes in two forms—K1 and K2. Vitamin K1 is found primarily in leafy green and cruciferous vegetables. Vitamin K2 is predominantly produced by bacteria and is divided into MK4 and MK13. These are found in some dairy products, pork, poultry, and fermented foods. Vitamin K2 may be more protective of bone.

## Structural Integrity

Small intestinal bacterial overgrowth (SIBO) is a common digestive imbalance I treat in the clinic. One factor that frequently contributes to SIBO is decreased intestinal motility. There are groups of nerves called plexuses that surround the intestine. When these plexuses are damaged, they do not function well. You can treat the microbiome until the cows come home, but if a component of SIBO is mechanical, it has to be addressed for SIBO to resolve. Gargling, singing, and using a tongue depressor to trigger a gag reflex stimulate the vagus nerve, contributing to good digestive motility.

Imbalances in the Structural Integrity Node often overlap with other nodes. For example, intestinal permeability, or leaky gut, a breach in the lining of the intestines, straddles both the Structural Integrity and the Assimilation Nodes. It's important to consider structure and function from a cellular level to the level of the larger systems, like the musculoskeletal system.

When structural integrity is optimized, optimal physical health is possible. Functions like movement, balance, strength, and cognition are optimized. We can hike, climb, dance, lift, move, and think at our best.

# Conclusion
## There Is Science and
## There Is Mystery

. . . . . . . . . . . . .

F OR NEARLY three hundred years, physics, largely based on Newtonian principles, helped us understand matter. Newtonian physics offers mathematical rules describing the motion of objects and math that allows us to look at the movement of fluids and curves. Sir Isaac Newton's principles continue to help us understand matter but are limited when applied to very small and very large scales. Still, Newtonian principles have been the foundation for understanding biology and medicine since the late seventeenth century.

Many of the world's leading scientific thinkers have been spiritual people who had some kind of belief in God or the power of the universe. Even for Newton—father of calculus, the three laws of motion, and the law of universal gravitation, and builder of the first telescope—science was but a small part of his spiritual quest. Gravity itself was a mystical subject because it involved forces unseen. Newton was an alchemist who seemed equally obsessed with ancient knowledge. Based on his writings, it is clear he believed a theological understanding of the world was compatible with science—and he went to great lengths to unify the two.

Charles Darwin advanced the science of evolution and biology largely through his now well-accepted theory that all living species descend from common ancestors through intrinsic processes of competition and selection. The convergence of Newtonian physics, Darwinian biology, and the conventional medical model has all but rendered the wisdom of healers and healing, traditionally the realm of women and women's work, obsolete.

However, there are limitations to what science and medicine can help us understand. Old theories of physics and biology fail to explain phenomena like healing from cancer, coming back from near-death experiences, or internal rotation during birth.

### Always Near to Mystery

What I miss most about no longer tending births is the loss of being in regular contact with mystery. One only need to witness internal rotation to realize the otherworldly forces at work during the birth of a baby. There are seven movements a fetus undergoes during labor. Internal rotation occurs when the baby's body and back of the head rotate from side to side to front to back to navigate the changing shape of the pelvis.

In part, internal rotation is pure physics: one shape efficiently passing through another shape. But there is mystery in it too. Physics offers no explanation for how a fetus "knows" it has to undergo a series of movements to navigate the bony pelvis and soft tissue of the mother. There is no assigned credit to the creator of this process. And, with such a tiny margin for error, how is it that it works flawlessly most of the time? Internal rotation exemplifies how the human body and nature transcend pure scientific explanation. Some of the "why" is inexplicable. Mystery remains.

Humans are desperate to understand. In matters of the body, we largely look to science for that understanding. Some people look to religion and others to astrology, but many people look to biology and chemistry. People want to know why they got cancer, why they can't have a baby, or why one person died from COVID when another person who attended the same party didn't get sick at all. There are limits to our scientific understanding and to what science can explain.

Not understanding, not being able to answer the question "why," can feel excruciating. If only you knew what to do differently to spare yourself, you would do it. But we don't always get to know. Not knowing propels us toward acceptance for that which defies reason and sense.

I've confronted mystery and the limitations of scientific explanation on more than one occasion in my own life: ruthless menstrual cramps; a spontaneous bleed when I was nineteen weeks pregnant with my son, and a long and complicated labor with him "even though" I was a midwife; a father with a brain tumor. Hands down, no questions asked, the largest mystery I live with is why Isabelle hit her head just so and died. Really? How does that work? "Blunt trauma to the head" of an otherwise thriving, beautiful girl, and, poof, she is gone? Physics and biology provide an explanation of sorts, but *why* Isabelle died will forever be a mystery to me.

I love science. I love understanding the mechanisms through which the body works, but like Newton and a long line of scientists and mystics both before and after him, I know physics and biology explain only so much. There are reasons other than just science for what happens in life, other forces at work, forces unseen. We know what we know for now, until information changes as the result of learning something new.

No one lives in your body except you, **which makes you the expert authority on you.**

———————

This is the work of science—to continuously pursue new information. The truth that has endured through the ages is that there is, and always has been, mystery.

## Interconnective Systems
· · · · · · · · · · · · · · · · · · · · · · · · · · ·

Quantum physics is revealing phenomena we cannot see as well as levels of interconnectivity previously not thought possible or understood. Interconnectivity transcends physical life and living beings. Quantum physics is a new frontier of science.

Considering our health from a systems perspective and practicing functional medicine is, in many ways, approaching health through an inherently feminine lens. Connectivity and interconnectivity are traditionally held feminine values and beliefs and, as such, stand to restore to health and health care so much of what is missing in conventional medicine as it is. The impact of such a restoration transcends individual health and extends to community and planetary health, all of which is sorely needed.

Functional medicine restores the focus of *collaboration* on the relationship between practitioner and patient, as opposed to the patriarchal, top-down, "doctor knows best" qualities that typically characterize relationships within the conventional medical model. Functional medicine practitioners practice *accepting*, as opposed to labeling a patient "noncompliant" when she doesn't do what she was "supposed to do." To get well within a functional medicine model requires *patience* as physiology is rebalanced.

While systems biology focuses on the interconnectivity within our bodies, quantum physics encourages our perspective to expand beyond our bodies, or matter, to include the nonmaterial world, or energy. The systems in our bodies are connected, and this connection transcends our physical bodies. We are connected to each other and all that surrounds us in intangible, invisible ways.

## An Invisible Web

Quantum physics explores the space that exists around physical matter. The smallest units of energy, or "quanta," are invisible to the naked eye. Quanta are often defined as meaning "packet" or "package." They are difficult to measure. They are simultaneously the smallest possible "thing" (matter) and a source for the largest possible energy (non-matter).

"Quantum plenum," meaning absolute fullness, is the term used to describe the space around physical matter. Quantum physics reveals that the space around matter is not empty; rather, it is an energy-dense medium full of potential. The space is primarily characterized by radiance, or light, and possibility.

From the quantum plenum, anything can emerge from something at any time. Imagine a pot of water on the stove the moment it starts to boil: a rolling simmer is a manifestation of the plenum. As I worked to get my head around these ideas, I consulted with my friend Karen Meritt, PhD, who teaches physics. She said to me, "Imagine dimensions in time and space with an energetic simmering that isn't driven by heat but instead by possibility." Endless possibility applies to our health, too, not just a pot of water being heated on the stove.

Karen demonstrated it to me this way: on my counter, she rotated a knife like a pinwheel. She described how Newton's work explains the forces moving the rotating knife. Quantum physics explains the space around the knife as it moves. We have to understand the knife, the matter, which Newton helps us do. Understanding matter is the scaffolding around which quantum physics emerges. Quantum physics is making sense of the space around the matter—in this case, the knife—and is revealing levels of interconnectivity not possible through Newtonian physics. Thus, science and medicine continue to evolve.

Here's the important part: The space around the knife appears empty, at least to most of us, *but it is not empty*. It is rich with energy and information and potential. Space is altered because of the presence of the knife, and the space around the knife is affected by the knife's presence. We can extend this understanding to our bodies: Our bodies are matter that arise in space. The space around our bodies is altered because of our presence. Within that space is a field of energetic potential; *we* exist within a field of energetic potential. When in a field of energetic potential, anything—and any amount of healing—is possible.

Why does matter, and the space around the matter, matter? Because matter changes. We change. The Earth changes. We are not separate from this change in matter, nor from the changes in the space around the matter. We exist on it and within it, and it is filled with infinite potential. This, I dare to say, is good news. On a planet that is warming, filled with viruses, and consumed by war, I feel hopeful when I recall we are filled with and surrounded by infinite potential.

Information is constantly being transferred between living things (the material world) and the environment. The brain and DNA transmit, receive, and interpret information from space, the field of energetic potential (the non-material world). The transfer of information between the material and non-material world yields a consciousness that transcends our tangible, physical bodies. Our ways of knowing go beyond that which we consciously think about. There is much to know about that which is not visible to the eye and the environment around and between us and the non-material world.

The space around matter presents the opportunity for you to move out of conscious thinking to subconscious awareness, in which the infinite potential of the non-material world is available to you. If and when you access it, how might it affect your health?

Some say we gain subconscious awareness through prayer, others say through presence. In his book *Becoming Supernatural*, Dr. Joe Dispenza advises practicing presence by "stopping yourself from thinking about the predictable future or from remembering the familiar past and simply unfold[ing] into this eternal vast space as an awareness—[to] no longer place your attention on anything or anyone material in this three-dimensional reality, like your body, the people in your life, the things you own, the places you go, and time itself. If you do that properly, you are nothing but awareness."

Being connected through a quantum field, an invisible web, changes ideas about self and other. There is no "self" and "other." There is no "me" and "not me." We are one. What affects one affects all. The fungi kingdom teaches us this. Coronavirus teaches us this. Lichen, part fungus and part algae, more than the sum of its parts, teaches us this. Everything is connected to everything. Greater things are born and understood through collective emergence.

Living with reverence for the interconnectivity of all living and nonliving things, the acknowledgment that we are not linear beings living a linear life, and that our three-dimensional reality is only a sliver of reality, prompts an enormous change in perspective. We shift from feeling isolated to part of community, from perceiving scarcity to abundance, from experiencing disease to health.

Quantum physics and expanding consciousness allow us to access limitless problem-solving possibilities and integrate theories of interconnectivity. We cannot solve problems we've created with the same ideologies and theories that created the problems in the first place. We need different ideologies and theories on which to base decisions, develop policy, and create new systems. Systems biology and functional medicine *are* the new systems for health and health care.

## The N of 1

Using evidenced-based research to substantiate clinical decisions is part of being a responsible health-care practitioner. But evidenced-based research is not the be-all and end-all of decision-making. There is tremendous value in considering the "N of 1."

N of 1 describes a clinical trial in which a single patient comprises the entire trial. You can think of your healing in the same way. Because you are biochemically unique, your experiences are what count in the trial-and-error process of creating more wholeness in your body and your life. The way you respond to a food, a supplement, a medication, or a toxin may very well be different from the way another woman responds to it. Your experiences are valid, even when a response to an intervention is unexpected.

There are observable patterns and universal experiences that can be leaned on when making health-care choices, but there is truly no way to know what effect any particular intervention is going to have on any one individual. I have made recommendations with the best intentions based on evidence and years of clinical experience only for a woman to experience the absolute opposite effect of what I intended. Who am I to say to someone that her experience is simply not possible or unrelated to the very thing I suggested she do? Anything is possible.

Which is to say, there is no one-size-fits-all medicine. For one woman, estrogen may decrease inflammation. For another, it may increase it. For one woman, decreasing her carbohydrate intake may reverse her insulin resistance, high cholesterol, and weight; for another, too few carbs may result in muscle wasting, depression, and weight gain.

Which is why you must participate in your own health care. You must advocate for yourself, speak up, and share your experience with your practitioners. For me, there is no way I can take good care of a woman without her communicating with me the cause and effect of what I suggested she try. She matters. Her preferences matter. Her experiences matter. As do yours. No one lives in your body except you, which makes you the expert authority on you. Don't give your power away to someone else who says they know what is best for you. Be your own health expert.

THROUGH THIS book, I intend to share some of what is currently understood about physiologic imbalances and how they manifest in the body. My intention is also to acknowledge that there are factors affecting our health beyond what is measurable and understood. Intangible, invisible, powerful, and mysterious forces course through us and around us. Our desire to understand may be the most intangible, invisible, powerful, and mysterious force of all.

Gratitude is the ultimate state of receivership.

I am so grateful for, and ever in service of, the mystery.

# Acknowledgments

· · · · · · · · · · · · · ·

'D HEARD people say "many hands touch a book" and "no one writes a book alone." I now know this to be true.

I feel the greatest honor to be entrusted with the physical, emotional, and spiritual care of my patients. Every one of you keeps me going, makes me smarter, and is such a source of richness in my life. Thank you for including me on your journey.

Bryan, there is not a dream I have pursued for which you haven't done all you can to support me. I am grateful for this support, your belief in me, and your flat-out stubbornness that has helped us through some of our darker times. I will never be able to answer your question, "Why is this our life?" but I'm glad we still get to share many blessings together. Thank you for helping make the dream of this book come true.

Aidan, etched in my memory forever will be the conversation we had walking in the woods when you explained the first law of thermodynamics to me as an answer to the question "Where did Isabelle go?" Your answer has been a well of peace for me. You are a beautiful amalgam of scientific mind, giant heart, warrior body, and wise soul. Thank you for bringing your perspective to these pages and to my life. I'm so lucky I get to be your mom.

To my family and Bryan's, thank you for your kindness and support through all the parts of this journey. Wit Bottle, I aspire to write as well as you when I grow up.

To my community, including my book and writing groups, who held me and my family with such astounding love through the unimaginable and who keep Isabelle's spirit alive. Your holding was our bridge to the present.

To the women on whose shoulders I stand—the nurses, the nurse practitioners, the midwives, the doctors, the healers who taught me how to tend to women with deep reverence for what is known and for mystery. I could not be the practitioner I am without you.

To Michelle and Ali of Soul Camp and Richelle of Purposeful Platforms. I had never experienced the sheer joy of creating something with other humans (other than children). Wow, was that fun. Thank you for pulling from me, shaping, and putting words and images to this vision. And to Ali S., the Freckled Yogi, I appreciate your earnestness and integrity. Thank you for filling in the blanks, for picking up where I leave off, for being the creative you are, and for understanding wellness from your being.

I deeply appreciate the integrity, professionalism, and conscientiousness of my team at Page Two, not to mention your careful tending to me and my ideas through an extraordinarily vulnerable process. Thanks for having my back and helping more women understand and access functional medicine.

Isabelle, we are tethered together forever. The absence of your physical body compels me to contemplate that which I cannot see and the notion that you are everywhere. I believe you *are* everywhere because there are moments, fleeting as they are, when I feel it to be true, and I am so thankful for them.

# Resources
## Keep Learning,
## Keep Growing

. . . . . . . . . . . . . .

FREQUENTLY RECOMMEND the following resources to women at the clinic. This list is by no means exhaustive. It is curated largely from my patients' experiences and my own, and I share it with you as a starting place for further learning and growth. I have organized the sources around themes for ease of reference, although some books may apply to health in several nodes.

IF YOU are looking to work with a functional medicine practitioner, I recommend starting your search on the Institute for Functional Medicine website, ifm.org. On the home page, there is a "find a practitioner" button, and you can enter your state, town, and zip code to learn about who is practicing functional medicine in, or near, your community.

## General
. . . . . . . . . .

### Books

*Accessing the Healing Power of the Vagus Nerve: Self-Help Exercises for Anxiety, Depression, Trauma, and Autism* by Stanley Rosenberg

*The Anatomy of Anxiety: Understanding and Overcoming the Body's Fear Response* by Ellen Vora

*Becoming Supernatural: How Common People Are Doing the Uncommon* by Joe Dispenza

*The Biology of Belief: Unleashing the Power of Consciousness, Matter & Miracles* by Bruce Lipton

*The Body Keeps the Score: Brain, Mind, and Body in the Healing of Trauma* by Bessel Van der Kolk

*The Disease Delusion: Conquering the Causes of Chronic Illness for a Healthier, Longer, and Happier Life* by Jeffrey Bland

*Eye of the Heart: A Spiritual Journey into the Imaginal Realm* by Cynthia Bourgeault

*The Field: The Quest for the Secret Force of the Universe* by Lynne McTaggart

*Food: What the Heck Should I Eat?* by Mark Hyman

*F\*ck Like a Goddess: Heal Yourself, Reclaim Your Voice, Stand in Your Power* by Alexandra Roxo

*In Defense of Food: An Eater's Manifesto* by Michael Pollan

*Mary Magdalene Revealed: The First Apostle, Her Feminist Gospel & the Christianity We Haven't Tried Yet* by Meggan Watterson

*The Myth of Normal: Trauma, Illness & Healing in a Toxic Culture* by Gabor Maté with Daniel Maté

*Perfect Madness: Motherhood in the Age of Anxiety* by Judith Warner

*Polyvagal Safety: Attachment, Communication, Self-Regulation* by Stephen Porges

*When the Body Says No: The Cost of Hidden Stress* by Gabor Maté
*Why Zebras Don't Get Ulcers* by Robert Sapolsky

### Online training
Gupta Program Brain Retraining: Limbic retraining for
  chronic conditions (guptaprogram.com)

### Accoutrement
Oura Smart Ring: If you like metrics, this little device monitors
  your sleep and other physiological measures (ouraring.com)

## Energy Node
. . . . . . . . . . . . . . .

### Books
*The End of Alzheimer's: The First Program to Prevent and
  Reverse Cognitive Decline* by Dale E. Bredesen
*Why Isn't My Brain Working? A Revolutionary Understanding
  of Brain Decline and Effective Strategies to Recover Your
  Brain's Health* by Datis Kharrazian
*Younger You: Reduce Your Bio Age and Live Longer, Better* by
  Kara Fitzgerald

## Communication Node
. . . . . . . . . . . . . . . . . . . . . . .

### Books
*Breath: The New Science of a Lost Art* by James Nestor
*The Functional Approach to Hypothyroidism: Bridging
  Traditional & Alternative Treatment Approaches for Total
  Patient Wellness* by Kenneth Blanchard
*The Role of Stress and the HPA Axis in Chronic Disease Man-
  agement: Principles and Protocols for Health Professionals*
  by Thomas Guilliams

*The New Our Bodies, Ourselves: A Book by and for Women* by
the Boston Women's Health Book Collective

*WomanCode: Perfect Your Cycle, Amplify Your Fertility,
Supercharge Your Sex Drive, and Become a Power Source* by
Alisa Vitti

*Women, Food, and Hormones: A 4-Week Plan to Achieve
Hormonal Balance, Lose Weight, and Feel Like Yourself
Again* by Sara Gottfried

*Women's Bodies, Women's Wisdom: Creating Physical and
Emotional Health and Healing* by Christiane Northrup

*Your Breathing Body* (audiobook) by Reginald Ray

**Websites and apps**

Calm app (calm.com)

Functional Fertility, Kalea Wattles (drkaleawattles.com)

Headspace app (headspace.com)

Insight Timer app (insighttimer.com)

## Assimilation Node

**Books**

*The Complete Low-FODMAP Diet: A Revolutionary Plan
for Managing IBS and Other Digestive Disorders* by Sue
Shepherd and Peter Gibson

*Digestive Wellness: Strengthen the Immune System and Prevent
Disease through Healthy Digestion* by Elizabeth Lipski

*Gut and Physiology Syndrome: Natural Treatment for Aller-
gies, Autoimmune Illness, Arthritis, Gut Problems, Fatigue,
Hormonal Problems, Neurological Disease and More* by
Natasha Campbell-McBride

*The Inside Tract: Your Good Gut Guide to Great Digestive
Health* by Gerard Mullin and Kathie Swift

*The Second Brain: A Groundbreaking New Understanding of Nervous Disorders of the Stomach and Intestine* by Michael D. Gershon

### Websites

"9 Ways to Use the Autoimmune Diet to Overcome Autoimmune and Hashimoto's Symptoms," Kharrazian Resource Center (drknews.com/autoimmune-gut-repair-diet)

Celiac Disease and Gluten-Free Diet Support (celiac.com)

Alexandra's Kitchen (alexandracooks.com)

## Biotransformation and Elimination Node

### Books

*Detoxification and Healing: The Key to Optimal Health* by Sydney Baker

*Toxic: Heal Your Body from Mold Toxicity, Lyme Disease, Multiple Chemical Sensitivities, and Chronic Environmental Illness* by Neil Nathan

### Website

Environmental Working Group's Clean 15 and Dirty 12 food lists (ewg.org/foodnews)

## Transport Node

### Books

*The Heart Speaks: A Cardiologist Reveals the Secret Language of Healing* by Mimi Guarneri (read anything written by Mimi Guarneri)

*What Your Doctor May Not Tell You about Heart Disease* by Mark Houston (read anything written by Mark Houston)

**Website**

HeartMath (heartmath.com)

## Defense and Repair Node

Book

*The Autoimmune Solution: Prevent and Reverse the Full Spectrum of Inflammatory Symptoms and Diseases* by Amy Myers

Podcast

*Solving the Puzzle with Dr. Datis Kharrazian*

## Structural Integrity Node

Books

*Better Bones, Better Body: Beyond Estrogen and Calcium* by Susan Brown (also visit her website, betterbones.com)

*Next Level: Your Guide to Kicking Ass, Feeling Great, and Crushing Goals through Menopause and Beyond* by Stacy T. Sims with Celene Yeager

*Roar: How to Match Your Food and Fitness to Your Unique Female Physiology for Optimum Performance, Great Health, and a Strong, Lean Body for Life* by Stacy T. Sims

## On Grief

Books

*Man's Search for Meaning* by Viktor Frankl

*Seeking Jordan: How I Learned the Truth about Death and the Invisible Universe* by Matthew McKay

*Signs: The Secret Language of the Universe* by Laura Lynne Jackson

*Where Did You Go? A Life-Changing Journey to Connect with Those We've Lost* by Christina Rasmussen

*Welcoming the Unwelcome: Wholehearted Living in a Broken-hearted World* by Pema Chödrön

*When Things Fall Apart* by Pema Chödrön

*The Wild Edge of Sorrow: Rituals of Renewal and the Sacred Work of Grief* by Francis Weller

# Glossary

. . . . . . . . . . . . . .

**adenosine triphosphate (ATP):** A coenzyme used as an energy carrier in the cells of all known organisms.

**antioxidant:** A molecule stable enough to donate an electron to a free radical, neutralizing its capacity to cause damage. Examples of antioxidants include glutathione, vitamin C, vitamin E, and beta carotene. Plants like onions, garlic, asparagus, and holy basil are rich sources of antioxidants. Berries, green tea, and dark chocolate are rich in antioxidants too.

**arthralgia:** Joint pain.

**autoimmune disease:** When a body's tissues are attacked by the immune system, expressing immune system dysregulation (impairment of the usual physiological function). Autoimmune disease occurs more frequently in women than in men because of the effects of estrogen on the immune system. Over twenty-three million Americans have autoimmunity. People with one autoimmune condition have a 25 percent risk of developing another.

**biotransformation:** The chemical modification of a compound made by an organism. Compounds modified in the body include, but are not limited to, nutrients, amino acids, toxins, heavy metals, and drugs. Biotransformation renders nonpolar (fat soluble) compounds more polar (water soluble) so they can be excreted. This prevents resorption of toxins into the renal tubules of the kidneys and the gastrointestinal tract.

**body burden:** The amount of toxins that have settled in a human body over the course of a lifetime.

**chronic inflammation:** Inflammation that lasts for prolonged periods of months to years. Chronic inflammation is the net result of a body's inability to clear the debris field.

**cytokine:** A secreted protein that allows for cell-to-cell communication. Interferons and tumor necrosis factor are examples of pro-inflammatory cytokines. There are anti-inflammatory cytokines as well. Interleukins can be pro- and anti-inflammatory.

**debris field:** Fragmented remains of dead or damaged cells or tissue cleared by a functioning immune system. Lack of clearance results in loss of tolerance and a burdened immune system.

**dysbiosis:** Imbalanced microbial communities in or on the body.

**elimination:** The process of getting rid of something. Within the context of detoxification, elimination happens through sweat, urine, and stool.

**endocrine:** Describes a type of hormone and the glands that make and secrete them into the bloodstream. Endocrine hormones travel through the blood and affect distant organs, including the pancreas, the thyroid, and the gonads, which are the ovaries in women.

**enzymes:** Substances that accelerate chemical reactions.

**food allergy:** A specific immunoglobulin E antibody response between an individual and a food.

**food sensitivity:** A specific immunoglobulin G or immunoglobulin A antibody response between an individual and a food. Food sensitivities can often be resolved by eliminating the food from the diet for at least ninety days. They often change over time.

**free radicals:** The by-products of energy production in the mitochondria as well as X-ray exposure, ozone, cigarette smoking, air pollutants, and chemical exposure. Free radicals have the potential to damage cells as they take oxygen molecules from healthy cells to stabilize themselves. The accumulation of free radicals is blamed for cancer, skin wrinkles, and aging.

**glycemic index (GI):** A way to measure the impact of food on blood glucose levels, on a scale from 0 to 100, based on how quickly the food raises blood sugar levels. Glucose (sugar) is calibrated to 100.

**glycemic load (GL):** A way to capture a more comprehensive picture of the glycemic impact of the diet as a whole. A GL is calculated by multiplying the GI of a food by the number of net carbohydrates (total carbohydrates minus fiber) in a serving. Low GL foods have a value of 10 or lower. They maintain stable energy for a longer period of time. Low GL foods include vegetables and whole grains.

**gut-associated lymphoid tissue (GALT):** A component of mucosa-associated lymphoid tissue (or MALT; see below). The gastrointestinal tract is a lymphoid organ, meaning it makes immune system cells. Other organs that do this are bone marrow and the thymus. The lymphoid tissue within it is referred to as GALT. The number of lymphocytes in the GALT is roughly equivalent to those in the spleen. The appendix is thought to be part of this system.

**Herxheimer reaction:** A short-term worsening of symptoms with the initiation of treatment prior to improvement, often observed in people being treated for Lyme disease. Ultimately, it is an increase in inflammatory proteins (cytokines) that the body then has to eliminate.

**hypertension:** Also known as high blood pressure, hypertension is an elevation in the force of the blood against artery walls. Blood pressure is determined by the amount of blood your heart pumps and the amount of resistance to blood flow in the arteries. The American Heart Association defines high blood pressure as a reading of 130mm Hg and higher for the systolic blood pressure, or a reading of 80mm Hg and higher for the diastolic measurement.

**hypothalamic pituitary-adrenal-thyroid-gonadal axis (HPATG axis):** The interconnected system of organs involved in hormone balance. The hypothalamus and pituitary are involved in sending signals to the adrenals, thyroid, and gonads/ovaries. The brain changes its signaling to the organs making hormones in response to perceived stress, a disrupted sleep cycle, blood sugar dysregulation, and inflammation.

**immune complex:** An antibody bound to an antigen. Immune complexes are part of a normal immune response. However, when immune complexes accumulate in the blood, they can cause autoimmune disorders, infections, and malignancies.

**intestinal barrier:** A functional entity separating the gut cavity from the rest of the body. It consists of mechanical elements like mucus and a tissue layer, elements that are part of the immune response involving antibodies (humoral) like IgA, immunological elements like lymphocytes and innate immune cells, and muscular and neurological elements.

**intestinal permeability (leaky gut or leaky gut syndrome):** This occurs when the intestinal barrier, which is impermeable when healthy, becomes permeable. When the intestinal barrier becomes permeable, substances that are supposed to be contained within the intestine "leak" into the bloodstream. Unrecognizable substances in the blood alert the immune system that something is amiss, triggering an immune response, leading to altered function and disease. Factors that contribute to intestinal permeability include changes in the microbiome, changes in the mucus layer of the gut, lifestyle, diet, and cell damage.

**-itis:** This suffix means inflammation, indicated in any word with this ending. For example: bursitis is inflammation of the bursa; tendonitis is inflammation of the tendon; capsulitis is inflammation of the capsule; colitis is inflammation of the colon; sinusitis is inflammation of the sinuses; or vaginitis is inflammation in the vagina.

**leaky brain:** The result of a compromise to the blood-brain barrier that results in it being permeable and allowing harmful substances to leak in.

**leaky gut:** See intestinal permeability.

**mast cell activation syndrome:** A condition that causes mast cells to release large amounts of chemicals into the body, causing allergy and a variety of other symptoms. Mast cells are part of the immune system that help fight infections and are involved in allergic reactions, including the release of histamine.

**metabolic detoxification:** A series of enzymatic processes that neutralize and solubilize toxins and then transport the toxins to secretory organs for elimination from the body. Metabolic detoxification is the collective work of the liver, kidneys, large intestine, lymphatic system, and sweat glands. It reduces the buildup of toxins in the body.

**metabolic syndrome:** The cluster of hypertension, hyperglycemia, excess body fat around the waist, and elevated cholesterol or triglyceride levels. Metabolic syndrome is associated with an increased risk of heart disease, stroke, and type 2 diabetes. It is typically caused by a Standard American Diet (SAD) and a sedentary lifestyle.

**methylation:** The biochemical process involving the attachment of a single carbon methyl group to a substrate. Methylation occurs in many biochemical pathways including phase II detoxification (see below), immune function, and DNA maintenance. Methylation of DNA represses gene transcription, controlling gene expression.

**microbiome:** The collective genetic material of the microbes—bacteria, bacteriophage, fungi, protozoa, and viruses—that live inside and on the human body. The microbiome moderates the interactions between food and the body, and it profoundly affects our mental and physical health. Whether a person develops a wide range of diseases, including cancer, cardiometabolic disease, allergies, or obesity depends largely on the organisms in and on the body. Specific diseases are being correlated with specific organisms living in the intestines.

**mitochondrion:** A specific structure found in most cells where cellular respiration and energy production occur. Plural: mitochondria.

**mucosa-associated lymphoid tissue (MALT):** The mucosa of the digestive, respiratory, and urinary tracts that contain lymphocytes (white blood cells that are part of the immune system).

**myalgia:** Muscle pain.

neuropathy: Weakness, numbness, or pain, typically in the hands and feet, resulting from nerve damage. Causes include B12 deficiency, diabetes, injury, infection, and exposure to a toxin.

neurotransmitters: Hormone messengers that affect mood, such as serotonin. Serotonin is the primary antidepressant neurotransmitter. GABA (gamma aminobutyric acid) is the primary antianxiety neurotransmitter. The majority of neurotransmitters are made in the gut, not the brain.

osteoporosis: When the creation of new bone doesn't keep up with the loss of old bone, resulting in weak or brittle bones prone to fracture or break. Bone mineral density is assessed using an X-ray called DEXA, typically taking measurements of the femur and the lumbar spine.

oxidative stress: The result of the imbalance between free radical generation and antioxidant defenses. Oxidative stress is implicated in the initiation, promotion, and progression of cancer, diabetes mellitus, eye disease, and neurodegenerative diseases.

phase I detoxification: The enzymatic transformation of fat-soluble compounds to water-soluble compounds. Phase I detoxification is generally carried out by a group of enzymes called the cytochrome P450 enzymes.

phase II detoxification: Biochemical processes that decrease the reactivity of water-soluble phase I products through enzymatic transformation. Phase II detoxification is carried out by enzymes such as UDP-glucuronosyltransferases (UGTs), glutathione S-transferases (GSTs), and sulfotransferases (SULTs).

phase III detoxification: The transport of water-soluble compounds out of the cells and the body through urine, sweat, and stool.

**pro-inflammatory cytokines:** A term used to describe chemical messengers that favor inflammation. Inflammation is the balance between pro-inflammatory and anti-inflammatory cytokines. Pro-inflammatory cytokines are made primarily by white blood cells. Examples are interleukin-1 (IL-1) and tumor necrosis factor (TNF). Pro-inflammatory cytokines stimulate fever, inflammation, tissue destruction, and sometimes shock and death. The production of pro-inflammatory cytokines is stimulated by infection, trauma, ischemia, immune-activated T-cells, and toxins.

**reactive oxygen species:** Chemical compounds that donate oxygen to other substances. Under certain circumstances, oxygen has deleterious effects on the body.

**small intestinal bacterial overgrowth (SIBO):** Occurs when bacteria from the large intestine ascend and enter the small intestine. Symptoms include, but are not limited to, bloating, abdominal pain (especially after eating), cramps, diarrhea, and gas.

**systemic yeast:** A spectrum of infections caused by different types of yeast including, but not limited to, candida. Systemic yeast infections can affect the blood, heart, brain, eyes, bones, or other parts of the body. Systemic yeast may be the root cause of constipation, depression, sugar cravings, itching (in the vagina, the ears, or the rectum), and skin rashes.

**tolerance:** Occurs when the immune system is unresponsive to substances or tissues that have the potential to induce an immune response.

**toxic load:** The accumulation of toxins and chemicals in the body, ingested or absorbed from a variety of sources, including the environment, food, drinking water, and personal care and household products. Toxic load is affected by genetic predisposition and a person's ability to produce enzymes necessary to process these compounds. Toxic load is strongly influenced by nutrition.

**toxicants:** Human-made chemical compounds with toxic potential.

**toxicity:** The degree to which a substance (a toxin or poison) can harm humans, animals, or any living organism. Acute toxicity involves harmful effects in an organism through a single or short-term exposure. Sub-chronic toxicity is the ability of a toxic substance to cause effects for more than one year but less than the lifetime of the exposed organism. Chronic toxicity is the ability of a substance or mixture of substances to cause harmful effects over an extended period, usually upon repeated or continuous exposure, sometimes lasting for the entire life of the exposed organism.

**toxins:** Poisonous compounds produced by living organisms. The primary source of toxin exposure for humans is food.

# Notes

. . . . . . . . . . . . . .

## Introduction

According to the Centers for Disease Control: "Chronic Diseases in America," Centers for Disease Control and Prevention, cdc.gov/chronicdisease/resources/infographic/chronic-diseases.htm.

The Institute for Functional Medicine was founded: "Putting Our Functional Medicine Vision into Action," The Institute for Functional Medicine, ifm.org/about/history.

## Chapter 4

gratitude also affords social benefits: Madhuleena Roy Chowdhury, "The Neuroscience of Gratitude and Effects on the Brain," Positive Psychology, April 9, 2019, positivepsychology.com/neuroscience-of-gratitude.

unhealed trauma may be the root cause: Irene Lyon, "Untreated Trauma: The Signs, Sources and Science," worksheet, irenelyon.com/wp-content/uploads/2019/03/Untreated-Trauma.pdf.

Trauma can cause a person to respond: J. Douglas Bremner, "Traumatic Stress: Effects on the Brain," *Dialogues in Clinical Neuroscience* 8, no. 4 (December 2006): 445–61, doi.org/10.31887/DCNS.2006.8.4/jbremner.

Early and developmental trauma: The result: Lyon, "Untreated Trauma."

## Chapter 5

Triggers affecting energy production include: Asa Hakansson and Goran Molin, "Gut Microbiota and Inflammation," *Nutrients* 3, no. 6 (June 2011): 637–82, ncbi.nlm.nih.gov/pmc/articles/PMC3257638.

Zinc may increase BDNF: Jing Du, Ming Zhu, Hongkun Bao, et al.,
"The Role of Nutrients in Protecting Mitochondrial Function and
Neurotransmitter Signaling: Implications for the Treatment of
Depression, PTSD, and Suicidal Behaviors," *Critical Reviews in
Food Science and Nutrition* 56, no. 15 (November 17, 2016):
2560–78, doi.org/10.1080/10408398.2013.876960.

## Chapter 6

Insulin resistance slows metabolism, increases: Ryan Raman,
"14 Natural Ways to Improve Your Insulin Sensitivity,"
Healthline, August 26, 2022, healthline.com/nutrition/
improve-insulin-sensitivity.

## Chapter 8

It provides direct chemical neutralization: Joseph Pizzorno,
"Glutathione!," *Integrative Medicine: A Clinician's Journal*, 13,
no. 1 (February 2014): 8–12, ncbi.nlm.nih.gov/pmc/articles/
PMC4684116.

Resveratrol improves vascular function, extends: Margherita Springer
and Sofia Moco, "Resveratrol and Its Human Metabolites—Effects
on Metabolic Health and Obesity," *Nutrients* 11, no. 1 (January
2019): 143, doi.org/10.3390/nu11010143.

It decreases liver fibrosis and steatosis: Forouzan Faghihzadeh,
Azita Hekmatdoost, and Payman Adibi, "Resveratrol and Liver:
A Systematic Review," *Journal of Research in Medical Sciences* 20,
no. 8 (August 2015): 797–810, doi.org/10.4103/1735-1995.168405.

Curcumin prevents liver injury by: Ishfaq Muhammad, He Wang,
Xiaoqi Sun, et al., "Dual Role of Dietary Curcumin through
Attenuating AFB1-Induced Oxidative Stress and Liver Injury via
Modulating Liver Phase-I and Phase-II Enzymes Involved in AFB1
Bioactivation and Detoxification," *Frontiers in Pharmacology* 9
(May 25, 2018): 554, doi.org/10.3389/fphar.2018.00554.

## Chapter 9

considers an elevated nighttime blood pressure to be: Mark C.
Houston and Lee Bell, *Controlling High Blood Pressure through
Nutrition, Nutritional Supplements, Lifestyle, and Drugs* (Boca
Raton: CRC Press, 2021).

Not all "bad" cholesterol (known as LDL): Stephanie Watson, "Can Good Cholesterol Be Too High?" WebMD, June 7, 2021, webmd.com/cholesterol-management/good-cholesterol-too-high.

About one in sixteen women: "Women and Heart Disease," Heart Disease, CDC, cdc.gov/heartdisease/women.htm.

Increasing heart rate variability decreases: Stefanie Hillebrand, Karen B. Gast, Renée de Mutsert, et al., "Heart Rate Variability and First Cardiovascular Event in Populations Without Known Cardiovascular Disease: Meta-Analysis and Dose–Response Meta-Regression," *EP Europace* 15, no. 5 (May 2013): 742–49, doi.org/10.1093/europace/eus341.

meditation can have long-standing effects: Glenn N. Levine, Richard A. Lange, C. Noel Bairey-Merz, et al., "Meditation and Cardiovascular Risk Reduction: A Scientific Statement from the American Heart Association," *Journal of the American Heart Association* 6, no. 10 (September 28, 2017): e002218, doi.org/10.1161/JAHA.117.002218.

Bergamot has been found to: Mirielle C. Nauman and Jeremy J. Johnson, "Clinical Application of Bergamot (*Citrus bergamia*) for Reducing High Cholesterol and Cardiovascular Disease Markers," *Integrative Food, Nutrition and Metabolism* 6, no. 2 (May 2, 2019): doi.org/10.15761/IFNM.1000249.

## Chapter 10

The conversation around immune system health: "Immune Fitness: Working Towards a Resilient Immune System," Nutricia Research, nutriciaresearch.com/immunology/immune-fitness-working-towards-a-resilient-immune-system.

Autophagy removes damaged cells coded: Sandra Yeyati, "Jeffrey Bland on Rejuvenating Our Immune System," Natural Awakenings, April 29, 2022, naturalawakenings.com/2022/04/29/397466/jeffrey-bland-on-rejuvenating-our-immune-system.

While we can't stop aging, we: Anna Aiello, Farzin Farzaneh, Giuseppina Candore, et al., "Immunosenescence and Its Hallmarks: How to Oppose Aging Strategically? A Review of Potential Options for Therapeutic Intervention," *Frontiers in Immunology*, September 25, 2019, doi.org/10.3389/fimmu.2019.02247.

The feed forward, self-amplifying loop: M. Cojocaru, Inimioara
Mihaela Cojocaru, and Isabela Silosi, "Multiple Autoimmune
Syndrome," *Maedic (Bucur)* 5, no. 2 (April 2010): 132–34, ncbi
.nlm.nih.gov/pmc/articles/PMC3150011.

One-third of the body's histamine: Datis Kharrazian, *Mastering
Functional Blood Chemistry*, lecture notes, delivered October
25–27, 2019, in Burlington, MA.

Considered to be the biologic door to: Alessio Fasano, "Zonulin
and Its Regulation of Intestinal Barrier Function: The Biological
Door to Inflammation, Autoimmunity, and Cancer," *Physiological
Reviews* 91, no. 1 (January 2011): 151–75, doi.org/10.1152/
physrev.00003.2008.

Daily meditation improves immune function: Richard J. Davidson,
Jon Kabat-Zinn, Jessica Schumaker, et al., "Alterations in Brain
and Immune Function Produced by Mindfulness Meditation,"
*Psychosomatic Medicine* 65, no. 4 (July 2003): 564–70, doi.org/
10.1097/01.psy.0000077505.67574.e3.

Exercise increases the immune system's: Ruth Sander, "Exercise
Boosts Immune Response," *Nursing Older People* 24, no. 6
(June 29, 2012): 11, doi.org/10.7748/nop.24.6.11.s11.

This significantly decreases exposure: Ifeoma Monye and Abiodun
B. Adelowo, "Strengthening Immunity through Healthy Lifestyle
Practices: Recommendations for Lifestyle Interventions in the
Management of COVID-19," *Lifestyle Medicine* 1, no. 1 (July 2020):
e7, doi.org/10.1002/lim2.7.

Rich in 2-HOBA, also known as: Jeff Bland, "Himalayan Tartary
Buckwheat: Meet the Next Superfood!" *Big Bold Health* podcast,
episode 20, January 29, 2020, bigboldhealth.com/podcast/
himalayan-tartary-buckwheat-meet-the-next-superfood.

Resveratrol improves vascular function, extends: Springer and Moco,
"Resveratrol and Its Human Metabolites."

It decreases liver fibrosis and steatosis: Faghihzadeh et. al,
"Resveratrol and Liver."

## Chapter 11

A study of post-menopausal women: Robert B. Wallace, Jean
Wactawski-Wende, Mary Jo O'Sullivan, et al., "Urinary
Tract Stone Occurrence in the Women's Health Initiative
(WHI) Randomized Clinical Trial of Calcium and Vitamin D
Supplements," *American Journal of Clinical Nutrition* 94, no. 1
(July 2011): 270–77, doi.org/10.3945/ajcn.110.

Vitamin K2 may be more protective of bone: Debra A. Pearson,
"Bone Health and Osteoporosis: The Role of Vitamin K and
Potential Antagonism by Anticoagulants," *Nutrition in Clinical
Practice* 22, no. 5 (October 2007): 517–44, doi.org/10.1177/
0115426507022005517.

## Conclusion

"stopping yourself from thinking about": Joe Dispenza, *Becoming
Supernatural: How Common People Are Doing the Uncommon*
(Carlsbad, CA: Hay House, 2019), 62.

## Glossary

A short-term worsening of symptoms: F. Angum, T. Khan, J. Kaler,
L. Siddiqui, and A. Hussain, "The Prevalence of Autoimmune
Disorders in Women: A Narrative Review," *Cureus* 12, no. 5
(May 13, 2020): e8094, doi.org/10.7759/cureus.8094.

Whether a person develops a wide range: C. Cullen et al. "Emerging
Priorities for Microbiome Research," *Frontiers in Microbiology*
(February 19, 2020), doi.org/10.3389/fmicb.2020.00136.

Specific diseases are being correlated: Joy Yang, "The Human
Microbiome Project: Extending the Definition of What
Constitutes a Human," National Human Genome Research
Institute, July 16, 2012. genome.gov/27549400/the-human
-microbiome-project-extending-the-definition-of-what
-constitutes-a-human.

# Index

. . . . . . . . . . . . .

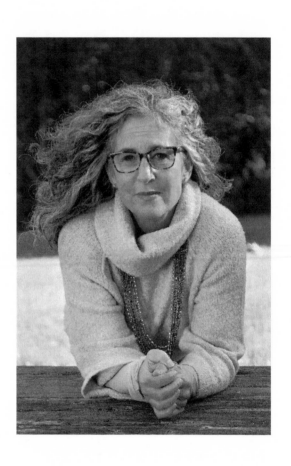

# About the Author

. . . . . . . . . . . . . .

CARRIE E. LEVINE, MSN, CNM, IFMCP, is the founder of Whole Woman Health. As a certified nurse midwife and an Institute for Functional Medicine certified practitioner, Carrie evaluates and treats the most common women's health concerns, incorporating gynecology and functional medicine.

Previously, Carrie practiced gynecology and functional medicine at the world-renowned Women to Women health-care clinic in Maine from 2006 to 2014. Prior to that, she practiced full-scope midwifery at Miles Memorial Hospital, now Lincoln-Health, in the beautiful mid-coast Maine town of Damariscotta.

Carrie is known for her ability to listen to and relate to women. For more than twenty years, she has been helping her clients identify personal health goals and break those goals down into attainable steps. She looks for the underlying causes of illness, seeking to connect the dots of seemingly unrelated symptoms and emotions. By supporting women in setting and achieving their own health goals, Carrie helps her patients thrive emotionally, spiritually, and physically.

Carrie earned a bachelor of science degree in public relations and women's studies from Syracuse University. She went on to earn her RN and MSN from Case Western Reserve University. Her certificate in nurse-midwifery is from the Frontier School of Midwifery and Family Nursing (now the Frontier Nursing University).

She is a member of the Maine chapter of the American College of Nurse Midwives, the Maine Nurse Practitioners Association, and the Institute for Functional Medicine.

# Join the Whole Woman Health Community

. . . . . . . . . . . . . . .

IN A CULTURE and society filled with resources about health and wellness, thank you for choosing this book. I hope it continues to be a valuable guide for you as you navigate your health.

My mission is to empower as many women as possible worldwide with information that will help them take good care of themselves and make sense of their health using the tools of functional medicine. It is also my aim to encourage deep and diverse conversations about health and healing.

If this book, through its specific chapters, general information, or stories, brought you value, please share it with a friend (or ten) and write a review at the online book retailer of your choice.

## Let's continue our conversation
. . . . . . . . . . . . . . . . . . . . . . . . . . . . . . . . . . . .

- Post your favorite passage from the book on your social media and tag me

- Find, follow, and engage with me online

    INSTAGRAM: @carrielevine.cnm
    FACEBOOK: facebook.com/carrielevine.cnm
    LINKEDIN: Carrie Levine CNM
    WEBSITE: carrielevine.com/contact

## Let's work together

- **Ordering copies for your organization:** Want to buy copies of this book for your organization? Contact me about bulk discounts and special offers at carrielevine.com/contact.

- **Speaking at your event:** Women's circles, keynotes, Zoom gatherings: whatever the event, I provide expert information that allows us to continue the conversation about health and healing.

- **Connecting with my Whole Woman Health clinical practice in Maine:** There is only one you, and an individual, tailored treatment plan addressing your specific needs and goals is the ideal. I provide care for women at every stage of their lives. I invite you to contact me for a consult to explore how you can benefit from our work together.

Made in the USA
Columbia, SC
16 January 2024

30547768R00188